A Guide to

The Vitamins

*Their role in health
and disease*

— A Guide to

The Vitamins —

*Their role in health
and disease*

JOHN MARKS

MA, MD, FRCP, FRCPath, Downing College, Cambridge

University Park Press
Baltimore

Published in USA and Canada by
University Park Press
Chamber of Commerce Building
Baltimore, Maryland, USA

Published in the UK by
MTP Press Limited
St Leonard's House
Lancaster
England

This book represents a revised and up-dated
text of an earlier book by the same author
entitled 'The Vitamins in Health and
Disease: a Modern Re-appraisal'.

ISBN 0-8391-0941-5
Library of Congress Cataloging Number 76-10048

Printed in Great Britain

Contents

PART THREE   TECHNICAL ASPECTS

Contents

The ABC of Vitamins

A

Oh fine and fat was Ralph the rat,
    And his eye was a clear cold grey.
How mournful that he ate less fat
    As day succeeded day.
Till he found each cornea daily hornier,
    Lacking its vitamin A.
'I missed my vitamin A, my dears',
    That rat was heard to say.
'And you'll find your eyes will keratinize
    If you miss your vitamin A.'

B

Now polished rice is extremely nice
    At a high suburban tea,
But Arbuthnot Lane remarks with pain
    That it lacks all vitamin B,
And beri-beri is very very
    Hard on the nerves, says he.
'Oh take your vitamin B, my dears!'
    I heard that surgeon say;
'If I hadn't been on standard bread,
    I shouldn't be here today.'

C

The scurvy flew through the schooner's crew
    As they sailed on an Arctic sea.
They were far from land and their food was canned,
    So they got no vitamin C.
For 'Devil's the use of orange juice',
    The skipper 'ad said, said he.
They were victualled with pickled pork, my dears,
    Those mariners bold and free,
Yet life's but brief on the best corned beef
    If you don't get vitamin C.

D

The epiphyses of Jemima's knees
  Were a truly appalling sight;
For the rickets strikes whom it jolly well likes
  If the vitamin D's not right,
Though its plots we foil with our cod-liver oil
  Or our ultra-violet light.
So swallow your cod-liver oil my dears,
  And bonny big babies you'll be.
Though it makes you sick it's a cure for the rickets
  And teeming with vitamin D.

E

Now vitamins D and A, B and C
  Will ensure that you're happy and strong;
But that's no use; you must reproduce
  Or the race won't last for long.
So vitamin E is the stuff for me
  And its praises end my song.
We'll double the birth-rate yet, my dears,
  If we all eat vitamin E.
We can blast the hopes of Maria Stopes
  By taking it with our tea.

C.H.A.

First appeared in
St. Bartholomew's Hospital Journal

Introduction

Throughout the history of mankind from primitive man to the present time, vitamin deficiencies have been a major cause of death and disease. Pellagra, scurvy and beri-beri have decimated armies, ships' crews and even nations (Figure 1). As late as 1925 the disease 'pernicious' anaemia caused by the absence of vitamin B_{12} within a person's body really lived up to its name.

Although there were isolated instances of recognition of dietary deficiencies even a thousand years ago, the importance of dietary factors in the genesis of these diseases was more widely recognized from the eighteenth century onwards and it was not until this century that the chemical structure of these factors was determined and the substances themselves synthesized.

As the science of biochemistry has developed it has been found that the clinical manifestations of vitamin deficiency follow derangement of multiple metabolic functions. The majority of the vitamins in fact form specific co-enzymes in various chemical processes but at least one is converted within the body into a hormone.

The commercial extraction and synthesis of the vitamins, which began mainly in the 1930s and 1940s, produced adequate quantities for a relief of vitamin deficiency diseases. The use of vitamins then became fashionable and dramatic cures were claimed for an ever increasing number of diseases. Subsequent careful observations have refuted these exaggerated claims. This in turn brought the negative reaction so typical of developments in modern therapeutics. Over the past few years editorials and government publications have repeatedly denied any value for the vitamins in industrialized communities.

This mainly nihilistic approach is now gradually disappearing as modern techniques of investigation demonstrate vitamin deficiencies in particular groups of people even in the most affluent societies. This has coincided with an increased number of careful experimental studies.

Soon after our passing *Streights Le Maire,* the scurvy began to make its appearance amongst us; and our long continuance at sea, the fatigue we underwent, and the various disappointments we met with, had occasioned its spreading to such a degree, that at the latter end of *April* there were but few on board, who were not in some degree afflicted with it, and in that month no less than forty-three died of it on board the *Centurion.* But though we thought that the distemper had then risen to an extraordinary height, and were willing to hope, that as we advanced to the northward its malignity would abate, yet we found, on the contrary, that in the month of *May* we lost nearly double that number: And as we did not get to land till the middle of *June,* the mortality went on increasing, and the disease extended itself so prodigiously, that after the loss of above two hundred men, we could not at last muster more than six foremast men in a watch capable of duty.

This disease, so frequently attending all long voyages, and so particularly destructive to us, is surely the most singular and unaccountable of any that affects the human body. For its symptoms are inconstant and innumerable, and its progress and effects extremely irregular; for scarcely any two persons have the same complaints, and where there has been found some conformity in the symptoms, the order of their appearance has been totally different. However, though it frequently puts on the form of many other diseases, and is therefore not to be described by any exclusive and infallible criterions; yet there are

Figure 1 Reproduction of part of an account of the effects of scurvy. Anson's voyage round the world (1740–1744) as recorded by Richard Walter. 626 of the 961 men died of scurvy rounding Cape Horn.

The purpose of this book is to review in a critical fashion the present state of our knowledge of the true value and importance of the vitamins. It attempts to provide a scientific basis for the effects of the vitamins by considering their biochemical and physiological functions within the body in relation to the disorders caused by their absence.

The book is primarily designed as an introduction to the subject for medical students, doctors and nutritionists. Although chiefly concerned with human problems certain aspects of animal disorders and animal husbandry are briefly considered as comparative biology has its relevance.

Part one

Nutritional Significance of the Vitamins

General Considerations

DEFINITION

The vitamins consist of a mixed group of chemical compounds. Their classification into a single group depends not on chemical characteristics, but on function. Vitamins are constituents of food; they are of an organic nature and are essential for the life and well-being of the animal.

Vitamins can be differentiated from the trace elements, also present in the diet, by virtue of their organic nature. It is more difficult to distinguish them clearly from certain other organic compounds in the diet which are likewise essential for health, as for example the essential fatty acids, which most people exclude from the list of vitamins. This distinction is largely based on the quantities of the material which must be present in an adequate diet. The vitamins are usually taken to include only those compounds which need to be present in low concentration (human requirements for compounds classed as vitamins at present are between about one microgramme and 100 mg daily). This sub-division of certain dietary essentials from the vitamins is thus rather arbitrary.

A further complication over the differentiation concerns the phrase 'constituents of food'. Certain substances which are still considered to be vitamins are synthesized by intestinal tract bacteria in quantities which are probably adequate for the needs of the body. Clear distinction is however made between vitamins and substances which are synthesized *within* the body. Ascorbic acid for example can be synthesized in the body itself by most species of animals, except when they are young, or under stress conditions. Thus ascorbic acid is *not* a vitamin under normal conditions for these animals. A similar but greater difficulty exists for vitamin D. Not only can this be synthesized in the skin of both animals and humans under the action of ultraviolet light, but both biosynthetic and dietary vitamin D act as prohormones in the body.

There is therefore no satisfactory current definition of a vitamin.

CLASSIFICATION AND NOMENCLATURE

The vitamins which have definitely been identified so far may be classified into two groups – the fat-soluble and the water-soluble vitamins.

When the vitamins were originally discovered they were isolated as essential constituents of certain items in the diet. At this stage, and indeed in the case of many for several years, the chemical composition of these essential factors was unknown. In consequence a system of designation of vitamins by letters developed. This system became complicated when it was discovered that some of the vitamin activity originally ascribed to a single compound depended on several compounds. In this way the designation of groups of vitamins appeared (e.g. the vitamin 'B' group). Additional chemical studies showed that variations in chemical structure occurred within compounds having the same vitamin activity but in different species. To overcome this a system of suffixes was adopted. The original simple letter system of designation thus became excessively complicated. Moreover, with the determination of chemical structure of the individual components, a letter designation was no longer required.

4

Trivial names were applied to the chemicals and irregularities which had grown up in the trivial names used in different countries have recently been overcome by an international commission. Nevertheless while it is now more logical to use these internationally accepted trivial names for the vitamins, certain of them are still known best by by their old letter designation. Table 1 lists the vitamins identified to date, together with their more widely used synonyms and the accepted trivial names.

Table 1 List of the recognized vitamins and their main synonyms. (Those in italics are the trivial names that are accepted.)

Letter designations	Synonyms
Fat soluble	
Vitamin A_1	*Retinol* axerophthol ⎫
Vitamin A_2	*Dehydroretinol* ⎬ antixerophthalmic vitamin
Vitamin D_2	*Ergocalciferol*
Vitamin D_3	*Cholecalciferol* calciferol, antirachitic vitamin
Vitamin E	$α, β, γ...tocopherol$ antisterility vitamin
Vitamin K_1	*Phylloquinone* phytomenadione ⎫
Vitamin K_2	*Farnoquinone*-menaquinone, ⎪
	multi-prenyl menaquinones ⎬ antihaemorrhage vitamin
Vitamin K_3	*Menaphthone* ⎭
Water soluble	
Vitamin B_1	*Thiamine* aneurine, antineuritic vitamin
Vitamin B_2	*Riboflavine* lactoflavine
Vitamin PP	*Nicotinamide* niacinamide
	Nicotinic acid niacin pellagra preventive factor
Vitamin B_6	Pyridoxine comprising *pyridoxol*
(as a group)	*pyridoxal*
	pyridoxamine
Vitamin B_{12}	*Cobalamin* ⎫
(as collective)	⎪
(pure substance)	*Cyanocobalamin* ⎬ antipernicious anaemia vitamin
Vitamin $B_{12}b$	*Hydroxocobalamin* ⎪
Vitamin $B_{12}c$	*Nitritocobalamin* ⎭
Vitamin B_5	*Pantothenic acid*
Vitamin M or B_c	
(as a group)	*Folacin* Lactobacillus casei factor
(pure substance)	*Folic acid* pteroylmonoglutamic acid
Vitamin H	*Biotin*
Vitamin C	*Ascorbic acid* antiscorbutic vitamin

THE UNIT SYSTEM OF MEASUREMENT OF VITAMIN ACTIVITY

Just as the initial absence of knowledge of chemical structure led to a letter system of designation, so in the early stages absence of data relating to the chemical nature of these new substances made it impossible to define dosage in terms of weight of active substance. The original examination for vitamin effect depended upon animal preventive or curative tests. This led to a system of units as expression of dosage, each unit being defined in relation to its effect on the animal.

The natural outcome of such a system was a series of different units established by different workers using different tests. It was only possible to corre-

Table 2 Summary of action of the vitamins.

Vitamin	Active Form (Enzyme or Hormone)	Function/Effect
Vitamin A	11-cis-retinal (visual purple)	Rod vision
	retinoic acid	Maintenance of epithelial integrity
Thiamine	Thiamine pyrophosphate	Aldehyde groups-transference of (Keto acid decarboxylase)
Riboflavine	FMN; FAD (flavoproteins)	Hydrogen (and electron) transfer
Nicotinamide	NAD$^+$; NADP$^+$ (transhydrogenases)	Hydrogen transfer
Folacin	Tetrahydrofolic acid (Tetrahydrofolic acid enzymes)	Formyl transfer ('C'$_1$ metabolism)
Biotin	Carboxybiotin (Biotin enzymes)	CO_2 transfer (carboxyl group transfer)
Pantothenic acid	Co-enzyme A (Transacylation enzymes)	Acyl transfer
Pyridoxine	Pyridoxal phosphate, acid decarboxylases, deaminases, transaminases, racemases)	Amino NH_2 transfer (and other functions in amino acid metabolism)
Cobalamin	B_{12} co-enzymes (B_{12} enzymes)	Isomerization, dehydrogenation, methylation
Vitamin C	Ascorbic acid, Dehydroascorbic acid	Integrity of intercellular substances. ? oxidation–reduction systems
Vitamin D	1, 25-dihydroxy cholecalciferol	Calcium and phosphate metabolism
Vitamin E	? tocopherol metabolite	Antioxidant particularly for lipids ? intracellular respiration, vascular integrity, central nervous system and muscle integrity. Normal fertility and gestation (all in animals)
Vitamin K	? 2 methyl-1, 4-naphthoquinone compound	? Hydrogen carrier Formation of certain clotting factors
Choline	Parent compound, bound forms, acetylcholine	Normal fat metabolism, compound of phospholipids, methyl donor for transmethylation

late these by reference to a standard preparation held by some central authority, or later by reference to a pure substance. To reduce the confusion internationally accepted units were established and these were subsequently defined in terms of weight of active pure substance, once this was available. Now that the composition of the vitamins has been defined, dosage is normally expressed in terms of weight and the unit system of measure is almost obsolete. The weight equivalents of the older international units are given under the individual vitamins.

BIOCHEMICAL FUNCTION

The biochemical function of several of the vitamins is now known. Thus, for example, the members of the B group are the main, or sole, component of co-enzymes. Co-enzymes may be regarded as components of an enzyme-prosthetic group complex which catalyse chemical reactions. Unless both enzyme and co-enzyme are present no catalysis takes place.

While the biochemical function of these listed members of the B group is now well known, less information is usually available on the biochemical function of the other vitamins except for vitamin D which is a pro-hormone. The main biochemical and physiological activities of all the vitamins are summarized in Table 2 (page 6).

Details of the chemical reactions and physiological functions of the individual vitamins are considered in the appropriate sections, but it will be seen that by virtue of these co-enzyme functions, vitamins occupy key and indespensable positions as catalysts in the metabolism of carbohydrates, fats and proteins, hence in the provision of energy within the body. A simplified version of the many functions of the vitamins in the complex biochemical reactions within the living cell is shown in Figure 2 (page 8).

CORRELATION OF CLINICAL FEATURES OF DEFICIENCY

It is at the moment difficult to correlate the exact physiological functions of the individual vitamins with the clinical manifestations of a deficiency. In the case of some of the vitamins clear and obvious correlation is possible, thus for example, night blindness occurs in vitamin A deficiency because this vitamin is part of the active light receptor in the rods of the retina.

However, such clear cut correlation is not yet possible for many other vitamins. It is to be hoped that the methods for cellular biochemistry, which have recently been developed, when applied to deficiency disorders, will help to answer some of these outstanding problems. At present it is indeed puzzling that the two vitamins which act on closely related metabolic processes within the Krebs cycle e.g. nicotinamide and riboflavine should exhibit such markedly different clinical signs and symptoms of deficiency.

DEFICIENCY DISEASES IN
THE MID-TWENTIETH CENTURY

In the world today, the explosive increase in population coupled with inadequate techniques of food production, is producing a mounting food deficit.

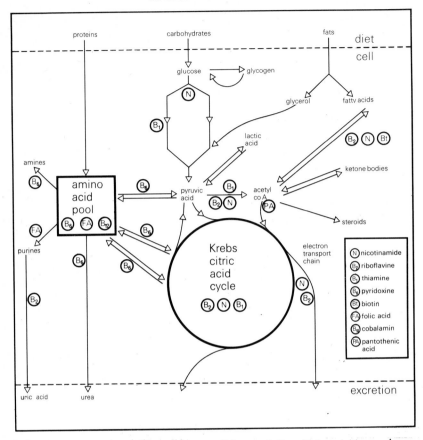

Figure 2 The importance of the vitamins in cellular metabolism. Main activities are shown in diagrammatic form.

Most of the countries of the world fall into two groups as far as food supply is concerned.

On the one hand there are the economically developed western countries, where there is food abundance. Approximately one-third of the people in the world live in these countries and enjoy a supply of food which provides on average about 3,000 calories per person per day. In the other group are the economically under-developed countries; the two-thirds of the world's population who live in these countries subsist on an average of rather less than 2,000 calories per person per day.

These two groups differ not only in the quantity of the food but also in its quality. The most significant deficiency is in protein and particularly in animal protein. In the developed countries the daily intake on average amounts to almost 40 grammes per person, while in under-developed countries the level is only one-fifth of this.

8

This difference between the developed and under-developed countries is unfortunately likely to increase over the coming years. For although the death rate is higher, the birth rate in the under-developed countries is about 40 to 45 per thousand annually, as compared with 17 to 25 thousand per annually in the developed countries. Thus the population increase is about 2·1 per cent annually in the under-developed countries and 1·3 per cent in the developed countries.

Thus calorie and protein deficiency, are the most important problems in nutrition at the present time. Vitamin deficiencies usually coexist with the protein-caloric deficiency. In the economically developed countries on the other hand inappropriate eating patterns can lead to bad nutrition resulting in vitamin deficiencies.

THE DEFICIENCY STATE

The presence of vitamins was originally recognized by the finding of classical signs of deficiency states. Attention therefore became focused on these clinical manifestations of vitamin deficiency. Administration of vitamins in these advanced deficiency states will reverse the majority of these clinical changes, but it is important to appreciate that not all such changes can be reversed. This is particularly true of those abnormalities which encourage fibrosis. A typical example of a disorder in which administration of adequate amounts of the vitamin will not produce reversal of the pathological process is keratomalacia (page 48).

After this early period of study of the vitamins in classical disease states, there was a swing in the opposite direction and claims were made for the effectiveness of vitamin therapy in many disorders. Subsequent controlled trials have shown that many of these claims were unjustified.

In consequence of the disappointment over these claims, and the general improvement in the nutritional status of the majority of people in the economically developed countries, a generation of physicians has now emerged who neglect to examine their patients for signs of vitamin deficiency. While the general population is adequately nourished, certain groups of patients will show signs of classical deficiencies (for example: Plates 7, 12, 13, 17 and 18 which were all taken during 1966). This aspect of the problem is dealt with later.

It is important to realise that the clinical signs of a vitamin deficiency are the end result of a chain of reactions. First there is a depletion of the vitamin stores, then a cellular metabolic change in consequence of the depleted co-enzymes. Only after these changes have reached the danger level do the classical clinical signs appear.

For example in a recent study in volunteers with vitamin B_1 depletion, no changes were found for the first five to ten days. Evidence of altered cellular metabolism could be demonstrated after ten days of depletion but the classical anatomical signs of vitamin B_1 deficiency were not obvious for about 200 days. In between the stage of biochemical abnormality and that of the classical signs there was a prolonged period of gradually increasing ill-health. Symptoms and signs during this phase were non-specific and included loss of body-weight, loss of appetite, malaise, insomnia and increased irritability (Figure 3).

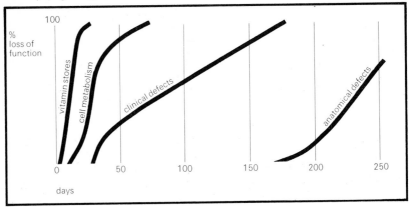

Figure 3 The stages in the development of a vitamin deficiency. Based on thiamine depletion in volunteers.

Altered cellular metabolism resulting from vitamin deficiency has only recently been studied to any extent. Not enough data exist about correlation of such biochemical changes with minor clinical abnormalities, nor do we know the end results of prolonged sub-optimal cellular activity. However, as a result of studies of this type many workers in the field of nutrition now believe that there has been too much pre-occupation during the past thirty years with the more obvious signs of clinical deficiency.

While accepting that the term 'optimal nutrition' is difficult to define, they consider this aspect is important for future studies in the field. Some aspects of 'optimal nutrition' are considered later (page 25). Experience in other diseases has shown the merit of treatment at the stage of cellular biochemical abnormality, rather than waiting for the final classical clinical signs. Thus for example it is now accepted that diabetes should be treated once hyperglycaemia is discovered, as this reduces the danger of diabetic arteriosclerosis and retinopathy. Accent has therefore been placed on some of the modern biochemical tests for distinguishing inadequate vitamin levels. These are considered in some detail later (page 169).

VITAMIN ANTAGONISTS (ANTI-VITAMINS)

While the alteration of the chemical structure of organic compounds frequently destroys their activity, minor changes in chemical structure on the other hand may not only destroy activity but also produce a direct antagonist to the parent vitamin.

A vitamin antagonist produces its effects by interfering with the conversion of the vitamin to its co-enzyme form or by displacing the co-enzyme from its combination with the protein part of the enzyme. Such an interference, particularly if it involves alterations in the enzyme itself, will not necessarily reproduce the effects of dietary deficiency of the vitamin. The difference between the presenting symptoms with dietary deficiency and with antagonists are particularly liable to occur when several enzyme systems utilize the same co-enzyme. The order in which the enzyme systems become disturbed may then differ and, in particular, will depend upon the binding potential of the antagonist at active sites on different enzymes. Although such antagonists have been used as a means of studying vitamin deficiencies, such results should be viewed or interpreted with caution.

Since co-enzymes play such an important role in cellular metabolism, antagonists have also been used for therapeutic purposes, particularly for treatment of cellular overgrowth as seen in malignant disease. Although such use is theoretically attractive, results in practice have not been encouraging apart from the use of certain anti-folic acid compounds in leukaemia in children.

Some anti-vitamin compounds occur naturally, for example avidin in raw egg-white; thiaminase in fresh raw fish. The mechanism by which these natural substances exert their anti-vitamin effect varies. Avidin, a protein substance, combines with biotin to render it unavailable to the body, whilst thiaminase splits vitamin B_1 into two inactive components.

Antagonists have now been found for most of the vitamins. They are considered in detail under the individual vitamins.

HYPERVITAMINOSIS

We are usually concerned with vitamin deficiencies, but it is also important to consider the possible effects of excessive quantities of vitamins within the body. For the water-soluble vitamins it is difficult to produce high tissue levels. By virtue of their water solubility, these compounds have a renal threshold and in consequence increase in blood levels above the threshold automatically results in loss of any additional vitamins in the urine. There is no evidence that the body is able to convert excessive quantities of vitamins into the co-enzyme form and thus elevate the intra-cellular active form above normal levels.

The only known example of toxicity to a water-soluble vitamin is the occasional hypersensitivity reaction which occurs when thiamine is injected (page 81).

With the fat-soluble vitamins on the other hand, excessive levels can be retained. Such excessive levels, if present for a long time, can themselves cause abnormalities. This is considered in some detail for vitamin A on page 49 and for vitamin D on page 59.

HEREDITARY VITAMIN DEFICIENCY DISORDERS

Most vitamins are converted in the body into co-enzymes which catalyse metabolic reactions in the presence of specific enzymes. Thus these chemical reactions depend not only on the presence of adequate quantities of the vitamins but also on an appropriate enzyme system. Enzymes are developed as a result of genetic factors within the nucleus and numerous examples are now known of altered enzyme activity due to abnormalities in the genetic code within the nucleus.

Among the genetic abnormalities now known to occur are some examples of an altered binding site for the co-enzyme. In such conditions abnormality of cell metabolism of the type seen in vitamin deficiency occurs, even though the co-enzyme is present in the cell in normal quantities. This has been most widely studied in the case of pyridoxine 'dependency' states (page 100).

There is, however, the possibility that other disorders may fall into this class and they are being studied at present with this in mind, e.g. Hartnup disease, a genetic variant of pellagra. The concept of vitamin dependency is a recent one and further developments in the field may be expected over the next decade. Genetically-determined abnormalities of the enzyme binding sites may explain the response of certain disorders only to vitamin levels well above those required for normal nutrition. Hereditary 'deficiency' states also occur for vitamin D. In these patients the abnormality is a failure to convert the precursor into the hormone form (page 56).

Causes of
Vitamin
Deficiency

For an active healthy life an individual must have a supply of each of the vitamins sufficient to meet the demands of the body. These demands vary from time to time depending upon changes in environmental factors. While some of these alterations are known, many are still the subject of conjecture. Vitamin recommendations proposed by official organizations attempt to include a margin to cover these unknowns. However recent studies in many countries suggest that the vitamin nutritional status of large numbers of people is not as adequate as was believed a few years ago. Some causes of vitamin deficiency are summarized in Table 3 and are discussed below.

INADEQUATE INTAKE IN THE FOOD

An inadequate diet may result from a general food failure in an area (e.g. due to drought) or from poor use of the available food by the individual.

Crop failure is rare in countries that are technically highly developed. On the other hand, failure of the year's crop due to droughts, flood or pests is still only too common in underdeveloped countries. Famine is still the largest single cause of general malnutrition at the present time. People affected show signs of multiple deficiency, including lack of calories, proteins and many of the vitamins. (This is considered in more detail on page 9.)

The general level of nutrition in technically developed countries is high and theoretically few, if any, inhabitants of such countries should suffer from vitamin deficiency. It must however be appreciated that, although the average diet in these countries is more than adequate in most respects, the tables

Table 3 Causes of inadequate vitamin intake.

Due to	Caused by
Primary food deficiency	Crop failure
	Food storage losses
Diminished food intake	Poverty and ignorance
	Loss of appetite
	Apathy
	Food taboos and fads
	Pregnancy sickness
	Dental problems
	Chronic disease
Diminished absorption	Absorption defect diseases
	Parasitic infections
	Malignant diseases
Increased requirements	Increased physical activity
	Infections
	Pregnancy and lactation
	Drug therapy
	Vitamin imbalance
	Rapid growth
Increased losses	Excessive sweating
	Diuresis
	Lactation

produced by health authorities probably overstate the margin of adequacy for the vitamins. Losses during storage and preparation of food, which are considered in detail on page 175, may be large.

While the average diet provides sufficient vitamins for the majority of normal people, various special factors affecting either individuals or groups of people can lead to suboptimal vitamin intake. Among these factors may be included:—

Poverty and ignorance

While improvements in the social services have reduced severe poverty many people are still too poor to buy enough food. Coupled with this poverty there is often gross ignorance of what constitutes a nutritionally adequate diet. Thus the money available for food is frequently frittered away on a diet which leaves much to be desired. Even when earnings increase the additional money is frequently not spent on food but, in order to satisfy a desire for social prestige, on bigger weddings, gaudy clothing and even jewellery. Indeed the diet may even deteriorate in times of greater prosperity as for example when the traditional unhusked rice is abandoned for the more refined but less nutritious polished form.

Lack of incentive

People living alone and particularly those suffering from chronic disease tend to eat food which needs little preparation. Thus items such as tinned meat, jam, biscuits and tea made with condensed milk figure largely in the diet. There is usually an excess of carbohydrates but the intake of protein and vitamins is often grossly inadequate.

Anorexia

Anorexia is a frequent precipitating cause of vitamin deficiency in a person whose previous nutritional status has been just adequate. Anorexia is common in the elderly, both in those living alone and in those in an institution. This anorexia results from listlessness, boredom and depression as a result of feeling unwanted. The loss of wider interests on retirement causes loss of appetite and may precipitate malnutrition in a person with a previous borderline nutritional status. This is particularly true of retired spinsters.

A further common cause of anorexia is an acute infectious disease. Even a relatively mild infection may cause a decrease in appetite or intolerance to food. In breast-fed infants such anorexia not only decreases their immediate food intake but may also lead to a more lasting disturbance. The infant fails to empty the mother's breast and milk secretion decreases. Thus at the time when nutrition is most important the food supply is least adequate.

Food taboos and fads

Many religious groups have specific and sometimes widespread food taboos. In some cases these taboos stem from sound public health ideas and benefit the community by reducing disease (e.g. avoiding parasite infected meat).

Many food taboos are without obvious foundation, have a deleterious effect on the general nutritional state of the community and persist in spite of changes in social structure.

Religious taboos not only specify particular items of diet but also define periods of total fast. The occasional day's fast, particularly in an otherwise well-nourished subject, may be beneficial rather than undesirable. However, more extensive fasting, particularly in groups whose nutritional status is in any case suspect, may do harm. Thus in Ramadan where fasting lasts for one lunar month each year no food or drink may be taken during the hours of daylight. Some of the specific food taboos relate to totem observance: some are based on the use of that particular species for sacrificial purposes. In some cases the food taboos have no direct relationship to religious beliefs but to a supposed deleterious effect of a certain food; for example in West Pakistan, it is believed that buffalo milk makes a person physically strong but mentally dull, whilst in the highlands of Bolivia any food containing animal blood is believed to make a child mute.

Many of these food taboos are confined to women, for the majority of the primitive communities were patriarchal societies. The lot of the pregnant woman is especially hard; for not only is she denied all the foodstuffs on the taboo list for women in general but, in addition to this, certain items of the diet are specifically forbidden during pregnancy in view of the supposed adverse effects on the foetus. It is thus scarcely surprising that, at a stage where requirements are highest, such low intake results in gross nutritional deficiencies.

In the western world similar problems exist, not so much as a result of taboos, but as a result of fads and fashion in dietary habits. Thus, for example there is the low calorie and vitamin intake of the fashion-conscious young and middle-aged woman attempting to slim. In the same age group the fads of the pregnant woman are well known. At the other end of the age scale, many elderly people develop food fads and the majority eat a far from balanced diet.

Dental problems

Dental caries and missing teeth can make eating uncomfortable and thus produce a very inadequate and distorted diet. This can occur in any age group but may play an important role in the elderly.

Apathy

There is often little incentive to prepare adequate meals and apathy towards food may exist. Thus the diet of those who live alone may become more and more monotonous and less and less nourishing. Impaired digestion is often associated with the apathy and this further lowers the nutritional status. This type of problem may be seen in the elderly, in the middle-aged bachelor or spinster living in a one-room apartment with or without adequate cooking facilities and in the teenager living alone for the first time.

Causes of Vitamin Deficiency
Chronic disease
Loss of appetite is frequently associated with chronic diseases. Therefore at a time when adequate nutrition is especially important (see below) there is an unfortunate mechanism which reduces the nutritional status by decreasing the food intake.

POOR DIGESTION AND ABSORPTION
Absorptive disorders
In the common absorption defect diseases (sprue, idiopathic steatorrhoea, fibrocystic disease of the pancreas, etc.) there is clear evidence of in-adequate absorption of the majority of dietary constituents. This applies not only to the main energy providing constituents, but also to the vitamins. In the majority of cases it is the fat-soluble vitamins that are least absorbed but deficiency of water-soluble vitamins has also been reported.

Parasitic infections
A specific effect of a parasitic infestation of the alimentary canal is seen in the case of infestation by fish tape-worm. This produces a deficiency of vitamin B_{12}.

The elderly ✄
In the aged several factors may contribute to impaired absorption and utilisation of the vitamins. These include defective mastication of the food, reduction of volume and acidity of gastric secretions, decrease of the secretion of digestive enzymes in the gastrointestinal tract and changes in the circulatory apparatus and organs.

INCREASED REQUIREMENTS
Physical activity
In Table 4 the recommended daily vitamin allowances for men under various conditions of physical activity are shown.

While the absolute values vary between countries, there is a general tendency to increase the recommended levels of thiamine, riboflavine, nicotinic acid and in some instances ascorbic acid as the level of physical activity rises. It is interesting to note that the figures given for the Soviet Union are particularly generous in this respect.

The evidence linking vitamin needs direct with the calorie intake is good for thiamine but less reliable for the other vitamins.

It must of course be appreciated that on a normal mixed diet, the measured need for thiamine or any other vitamin should be met by the larger quantities of food consumed.

Rapid growth
As might be anticipated from their metabolic functions there is clear evidence, both from animal experiments and human observations, that vitamin requirements are increased during periods of rapid growth.

17

Table 4 Recommended dietary allowance for men (25–26 years) under various conditions of physical activity. Differences demonstrated by reference to values from selected countries.

Vitamin		GB	West Germany	USSR
B$_1$mg	Sedentary	1·0	1·7	—
	Moderately active	1·2	2·2	2·0
	Active	1·4	2·5	2·5
	Very active	1·7	2·9	3·0
B$_2$mg	Sedentary	1·5	1·8	—
	Moderately active	1·8	1·8	2·5
	Active	2·1	1·8	3·0
	Very active	2·6	1·8	3·5
Nic.acid mg	Sedentary	10	—	—
	Moderately active	12	—	15
	Active	14	—	20
	Very active	17	—	25
C mg	Sedentary	20	75	—
	Moderately active	20	75	70
	Active	20	75	100
	Very active	20	75	120

Early animal observations showed that normal growth could only take place when the vitamin intake was adequate. The commercial background of animal husbandry has subsequently ensured that vitamin levels for animal growth have been fully studied. As a result literature relating to animal vitamin needs normally specifies 'optimum' level rather than 'adequate' intake (page 25). Less accurate information is however available on the vitamin requirements for growth of children. Most authorities agree however that the need in children is relatively higher than the need in adults, particularly considered on a body-weight or food intake basis.

Infections

For generations it has been appreciated that malnutrition makes men more susceptible to infections. While circumstantial evidence is plentiful, clear experimental evidence implicating specific nutritional deficiencies is still largely lacking, particularly for infections in humans. The relationship between infections and general malnutrition is indeed synergistic, for infections can aggravate malnutrition, which in its turn weakens resistance to infection. The result may therefore be more serious to the host than the additive effect of the two acting independently. This synergistic effect is seen at its worst in the high mortality in young children in developing countries. Existing data suggest that these considerations apply to bacterial (e.g. tuberculosis), viral (e.g. measles) and parasitic infections. Deficiencies of vitamin A and C are the most likely to predispose to infections. A typical example of additive effects between infection and vitamin A deficiency is the frequency

18

with which keratomalacia is precipitated by an intercurrent infection, even when the diet remains constant.

Evidence suggests that the following factors may play a part in the reduced resistance to infections in vitamin deficiency; reduced antibody formation, reduced phagocytic activity, decreased levels of protective enzymes (e.g. lysozymes), and reduced tissue integrity particularly of the skin and mucous membranes.

Whilst evidence about the part played by inadequate vitamin intake in the development of infections is on the whole based upon very little data, there is ample evidence of the part that infections can play in the precipitation of true vitamin deficiencies. For example it has been known for many years that children with meningococcal meningitis, diarrhoea, febrile tuberculosis, measles and many other acute infections, may develop keratomalacia which may end in blindness. While these overt signs of vitamin deficiency are more likely to be seen in groups of people in whom the vitamin intake is low, observations in patients of good nutritional status with infections have shown a decreased level of vitamin A as the infection progresses.

Cases have been reported of overt scurvy appearing in children who have suffered from a febrile illness. Recently experimental work following vaccination has shown that this infection, even in healthy subjects, can result in a marked decrease in the vitamin C level in the body.

Prisoners in the far east during the second world war who were on a thiamine deficient diet, but who showed no overt signs of this deficiency, frequently developed the symptoms and signs of beri-beri following infectious diarrhoea.

Pregnancy and lactation ✗

In numerous investigations marked reductions of the blood levels of vitamin A, nicotinic acid, pyridoxine, vitamine B_{12} and ascorbic acid have been found in pregnant women. Even now, however, we know little about the precise vitamin requirements during pregnancy and lactation. The most careful studies are probably those on pyridoxine, the results of which suggest that the pregnant woman needs approximately 10 mg of the vitamin to maintain normal function compared with an estimate of about 2 mg in normal women.

The paucity of information of the exact needs in pregnancy and lactation may be judged from the marked differences in the amounts that are recommended in various countries as compared with those recommended for normal women for the same countries. However, although individual figures vary, an increased level is generally recommended.

Drug therapy

During the past few years drug-induced vitamin deficiencies have become more prevalent. Among the most common are the vitamin B complex deficiencies arising during treatment with the broad-spectrum antibiotics.

The exact aetiology is still far from clear and results of treatment after symptoms and signs become obvious have often been rather unpromising. The present evidence suggests that vitamin B complex supplementation should be given whenever treatment with broad-spectrum antibiotics is likely to continue for more than two to three days. This is particularly desirable where a low vitamin level is suspected at the start of antibiotic therapy, as may be the case in the elderly.

Pyridoxine is one vitamin that appears to be particularly vulnerable to depletion during drug therapy. Thus clinical pyridoxine deficiency has for example been reported during isoniazid and penicillamine therapy and with the use of steroid contraceptives.

The administration of oral contraceptives appears to reduce the plasma levels of all the water soluble vitamins tested though the clinical significance of this is not clear.

Other components of the diet

Vitamin requirements are related to the dietary intake of those substances in whose metabolism they are involved. Thus, for example, the thiamine requirement is increased by high carbohydrate intake while a diet rich in protein requires more pyridoxine. The protein intake appears to influence also the riboflavine requirement, since the retention of this vitamin seems to be poorer with low protein intake.

The requirement for vitamin E varies directly with the amount of unsaturated fatty acids ingested. One specific instance has been found of an individual amino acid affecting vitamin requirements; leucine found in high content in millet increases the requirement for nicotinic acid. This is particularly important in India where millet forms a large proportion of the diet. Avidin, a protein contained in raw white of egg, which combines with biotin may precipitate a biotin deficiency.

Some raw fish contains a thiamine-splitting enzyme, thiaminase, and in those countries where large amounts of fish are eaten raw, thiamine deficiency may occur. Some bacteria, e.g. *Bacillus thiaminolyticus*, are also capable of breaking down thiamine. It is reported that some 3 per cent of Japanese show a thiamine deficiency due to infection with this bacillus.

The influence of other vitamins

From experimental studies in animals it is known that the requirement of one vitamin may be influenced to a considerable extent by the level of the other vitamins in the experimental diet. Thus, for example, in lambs it is possible to precipitate rickets by giving a diet with minimal but just adequate vitamin D and increasing the level of carotene. Equally a deficiency of one vitamin may precipitate the deficiency of another—for example ascorbic acid is needed in the conversion of folic acid to folinic acid and therefore vitamin C deficiency may be accompanied by signs of folic acid deficiency.

The extent to which these interactions are relevant to human nutrition is still far from clear. Nevertheless experience with grossly abnormal diets in prisoner of war camps suggests that vitamin interactions of this type may also play a part in human malnutrition.

Excessive losses

Most of the water soluble vitamins are present in the body excretions e.g. urine, sweat.

In some cases the extent of the loss appears to be related directly to the volume of the excretion.

The importance of such losses in the overall vitamin balance of the body has been studied very little. Existing data suggest however that losses in the sweat during physical activity in hot climates is sufficient to raise the requirements under such conditions.

Vitamin Adequacy
of the
Average Diet

Considerable differences of opinion exist among nutritionists and physicians concerning the adequacy of the average diet in terms of vitamin content. There is a general feeling that the diet of people living in most industrialized countries is completely adequate for the supply of all nutrient substances including vitamins. On the other hand some experts believe that a significant proportion of the normal population of industrialized countries may have reduced vitamin reserves.

Probably the main problems are the definition of an 'average diet' and of a 'normal person'. Typical well-balanced diets as given in nutrition handbooks do indeed provide adequate amounts of nutrients. It is necessary to establish how generally a well-balanced diet is actually consumed. Recent surveys of selected groups of 'normal' subjects in several countries have demonstrated clear biochemical evidence of multiple vitamin deficiencies. It must however be stressed that the majority of normal subjects show no clinical evidence of a vitamin deficiency. The reports of frank vitamin deficiency that are still being published in the medical journals of the Commonwealth, Europe and the United States show that certain segments of even affluent societies may be grossly vitamin deficient. Moreover recently reported findings, that some 19 per cent of autopsy hearts from patients with a clinical diagnosis of arterio-sclerosis and cardiac decompensation, showed the characteristic changes of beri-beri lead one to question the validity of our present clinical examinations for vitamin deficiency. Numerous surveys have indeed been undertaken to determine whether the 'normal' diet is adequate. The majority of these surveys may be criticized on the following bases:

1 Many are concerned with an *average* of the overall food usage, i.e. the total quantity of food consumed divided by the total population number. Such surveys take no account of the great variability in the eating habits of groups or individuals. Where studies have been undertaken of individual food consumption, it is found that some people are consuming well below the calculated average.

2 The amount of food entering the kitchen does not give a true representation of the food that is actually consumed. It takes no account of the amount of food that is wasted, either during preparation or from the table. The extent of this wastage is easily seen from an examination of the swill bucket.

3 The nutrient content of the diet is normally calculated from published tables, but many of these are based on older methods of analysis. Re-examination using modern analytical techniques shows their inaccuracy but more extensive data is needed. A number of recent studies have shown that the older figures are too high, even for fresh food.

4 Food suffers considerable but variable loss of nutrients, particularly vitamins, on the way from the garden to the gullet. The reason for these losses and their extent under varying circumstances and for various vitamins is considered in more detail on page 176.

5 The requirement is modified by other food factors (see page 20).

6 Most of these stated requirements are concerned with 'adequate' re-

quirements, rather than with optimal amounts which would allow full and efficient total activity.

On the basis of evidence available at present it must be concluded that healthy individuals taking an above average, or average, balanced diet will not suffer from any vitamin deficiency. They will probably receive sufficient of most of the vitamins even for periods of marked activity or stress. Even so there are individuals within the general population, who for one reason or another (pages 14 to 21), whilst otherwise normal are receiving a below average diet. Evidence gained over the past years suggests that many such people are sub-optimal in respect to their vitamin nutrition, and that, in a proportion, frank vitamin deficiency exists. The extent of this problem in the 'normal' population is however still a matter for dispute and the problem will only be resolved when further studies using the best modern techniques are undertaken.

OPTIMUM VITAMIN INTAKE

Several examples are available of improved performance in animals from dietary levels of vitamins in excess of the minimum required for apparent health. Thus, for example:

1 Clinical. Signs of a deficiency of vitamin B_6 have never been observed under field conditions in piglets. Xanthurenic acid excretion after tryptophan load may however be used as a biochemical index of inadequate pyridoxine intake.

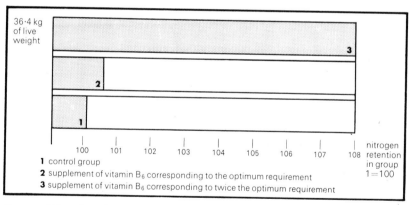

Figure 4 Effect of pyridoxine supplements on nitrogen retention in growing pigs.

In growing pigs, which have received rations of protein-concentrates, barley and tapioca meal but with no added pyridoxine, there was biochemical, but no clinical evidence of inadequate pyridoxine supply. However, addition of pyridoxine to the ration allowed up to 20 per cent more nitrogen retention from the diet. A typical experimental observation is shown in Figure 4.

2 In growing calves extensive work has been undertaken on vitamin A

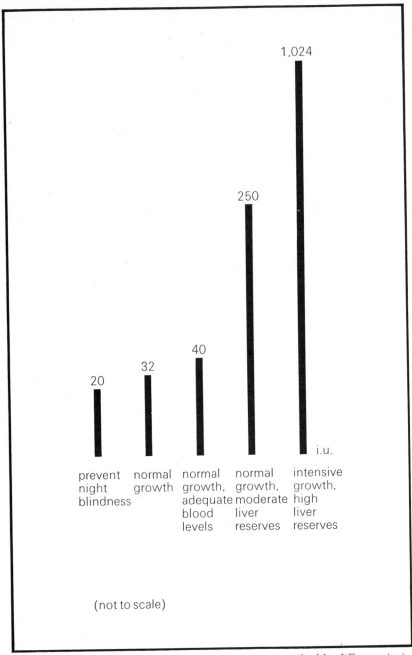

Figure 5 Estimates of the vitamin A requirements of calves as judged by different criteria (i.u. per day).

requirements. Some of this data is shown diagrammatically in Figure 5. It will be seen that while the minimum requirement to prevent night blindness is approximately 20 i.u./kg. body-weight per day some 40 times this level is necessary for intensive growth with very high liver reserves. The optimal value for calves probably lies somewhere between these two extremes.

3 In chicks, the average growth on various dietary intakes of vitamin B_6 is shown in Figure 6. A dose of 50 mg per 100 g feed is adequate to prevent any clinical evidence of pyridoxine deficiency, nevertheless, a fourfold increase of this dose produces a marked additional rate of growth.

Table 5 Vitamin requirements for various animal species extrapolated on a body-weight basis to a 70 kg man. Compared with recommended human levels. USA data has been used throughout.

	Vitamin A i.u	Vitamin D i.u.	Vitamin B_1 mg	Vitamin B_2 mg	Nic.acid mg	Vitamin B_6 mg	Vitamin C mg
Man	5000	—	1·4	1·6	18	2·0	45
Cow (milking)	7500	450	—	—	—	—	—
Horse (working)	6000	450	3·75	3·0	15	3·75	—
Pig (sow)	10,500	1050	2·25	6·0	22·5	3·75	—
Dog	25,500	450	6·0	3·0	16·5	1·5	—
Hen (laying)	12,000	1300	5·0	5·0	90	7·4	—

In Table 5 the vitamin requirements for various animal species have been extrapolated to the human on a standard 70 kg body-weight basis. The levels are compared with those recommended for human use in the most recent report from the United States since the animal data are also derived from American sources.

It is fully appreciated that such extrapolation is open to criticism on many counts. Nevertheless it is interesting to note that, with the possible exception of nicotinic acid, the recommended levels for man are well below those for these other important species on a weight basis.

While the concept of optimal dietary intakes is now well established for animals, the present available data do not allow us to to establish similar optimal levels for the human. Nevertheless there would seem to be a need for further investigation of this problem. In particular the effect of common stresses (infection, physical activity, rapid growth, etc.) on the dietary requirements should be studied with care. Vitamin supplementation of the diet is now not an expensive procedure. Our lack of knowledge of the best intake per day is shown conclusively by the wide range recommended in different countries.

The main problem for assessment of the appropriate dietary level for any vitamin in the human diet is the determination of the significance of different criteria. The first effect of a vitamin deficiency is a reduced tissue level or reserve. At a variable, but at present ill-defined level of tissue vitamin depletion the biochemical function is reduced or lost. Once the abnormality in

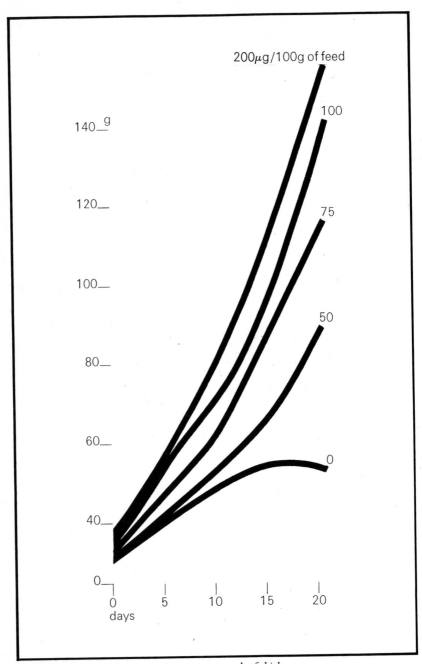

Figure 6 Effect of pyridoxine supplements on growth of chicks.

enzyme function reaches a critical level clinical evidence of the vitamin deficiency appears.

In humans, levels have been established which will guarantee that clinical signs of deficiency do not appear. In animals it has been shown that increasing the levels above these values and approaching those that give full tissue loading improves health and performance. Similar data is still not available in the human.

If we may judge by animal experience, and in the case of the vitamins, animal data is often a reasonably reliable guide to human needs, supplementation to an optimal intake would probably result in increased performance and reduced incidence of illness.

Vitamin Problems in Underprivileged Countries

Recent evidence suggests that the vitamin levels of certain groups of people in industrialized countries are inadequate. However the extent of these vitamin deficiencies is minimal compared with the major nutritional problems which exist in many parts of the world.

CAUSE

The cause of gross malnutrition in any particular community usually involves a number of factors. Since these are commonly inter-related a vicious circle may be established. Nevertheless it is possible to define four main general causes for this widespread problem.

1 *Poor climatic conditions*

In some areas of the world adequate food can not be produced to support the local population due to the poor climatic conditions. In many of these areas population density is in fact not excessive when compared with industrialized countries. The possibilities of producing food locally are, however, so limited that even a low population density cannot be nourished. These areas include the

Polar regions Alaska, Lapland, North of Canada.

Deserts in Africa – parts of Egypt and all countries bordering on the Sahara Desert; in America – parts of Mexico, Peru and Chile; in Asia – the desert lands of the Middle East.

Tropical rain forests in Africa – much of the equatorial region; in America – parts of central America, Brazil, Peru; in Asia – the equatorial regions of South East Asia.

These countries must depend upon a food supply from outside, which in turn often has to be paid for by exports from limited local resources, e.g. minerals, cocoa, palm oil, petrol, etc. Thus variations in the world price of these commodities automatically reflects on the nutritional status of the community. The only feasible method of achieving rapid improvement in the situation is by the provision of food including vitamin supplements cheaply from other countries. The deficiency is usually more extensive than merely the absence of vitamins and work is proceeding on the development of special protein-rich foods derived from natural resources. However, the vitamin content of these foods is usually low and requires supplementation.

2 *High population density with low economic status*

In many areas of the world the growth of population has been both extensive and rapid. In these areas, even given ideal soil and weather conditions, inadequate natural resources exist to feed the whole population.

In the industrialized countries the economic status is such that the difference between the amount of food produced locally and that required for adequate nutrition can be overcome by appropriate food imports. In these countries the general level of nutrition is high and vitamin deficiency states are found only in particular groups of people.

In those countries, on the other hand, which are less developed the general economic situation is poor and insufficient foreign currency is available to allow importation of food to bridge the nutrition gap for the whole population. Malnutrition in these countries is the rule rather than the exception. In such territories inefficient methods of farming are used and yields are only a fraction of the theoretical maximum.

Most of the countries in which the high density of population is a major factor in malnutrition are to be found in the sub-tropical and tropical regions of Asia.

While the development of better methods of farming in these areas will reduce the problem it is unlikely that these will keep pace with the rate of population growth. Neither would distribution of wealth and resources, as some ideologists would have us believe, solve the problem.

Extrapolation of the world population statistics suggests that this will become an increasing and widening problem over the next decade. The available utilizable land mass is incapable of yielding adequate food to provide a reasonable nutritional level for this increased world population, even if yields are brought to a maximum and distribution is even. The vitamin deficiency part of this problem can be overcome by the use of synthetic products. An adequate calorie and protein intake could only be achieved by revolutionary methods of food harvesting from land or sea or by a radical birth control programme.

3 Food taboos

Although not confined to the under-privileged countries, food taboos are found more commonly there. Based upon tribal or religious customs, many were also originally based, although perhaps unwittingly, on sound scientific factors (e.g. avoidance of helminth infected food, encouragement of the fishing industry, etc.). Once they were firmly established by custom or decree, the basic reason was often forgotten. Changes are difficult to achieve when the raison d'être has gone. The problem of these food taboos is considered in more detail on page 15.

4 Inadequate facilities for health and nutrition education

One of the most difficult problems facing the developing countries is that of re-educating people to take advantage of new facilities, including not only those for food production, food handling and storage, but also for the preparation and use of unusual foods and of dietary supplements. The problem arises partly from inadequate numbers of trained personnel, but partly from the laissez faire attitude which is so common in hot climates. Programmes for financial help from the industrialized countries can only succeed if they are coupled with corresponding programmes for re-education.

It must be appreciated that while the theoretical causes of malnutrition in these territories can be stated in isolation, in practice more than one factor is usually involved in any particular country. Thus for example in most of these territories there are areas which are capable of high food yield and other arid areas where food production would only be possible as a result of a long term programme to provide adequate water. Experimental methods under trial include reafforestation to encourage rainfall, river dams and artificial irrigation techniques.

THE NATURE OF THE VITAMIN DEFICIENCIES THAT OCCUR IN DEVELOPING COUNTRIES

In spite of the widespread general malnutrition, classical signs of florid vitamin deficiencies are not as widespread as might be anticipated and instead rather bizarre deficiency signs are usually encountered. This is probably due to the simultaneous existence of multiple dietary deficiencies – calorie, protein, vitamin and mineral.

Although several surveys have been undertaken both by national and by international bodies, considerable work still needs to be done before the nature and extent of malnutrition can be fully known. When we come to studies of individual vitamin deficiencies in many of these areas, still less is known and several years will probably elapse before a clear picture emerges.

Techniques for vitamin assays which can be correlated with clinical signs are only now reaching a stage where some measure of accuracy can be expected. Such techniques are however more suited to the well equipped research laboratory than to field surveys. Some of the techniques used previously are now known to be unreliable and therefore earlier reports can only be regarded as providing a rough guide.

It is apparent from the recent vitamin surveys that there is widespread evidence of multiple vitamin deficiencies as judged by biochemical estimations. The significance of the correlation of these biochemical determinations with clinical states is considered in more detail on page 170. It seems likely that classical signs of deficiency of single vitamins or groups of vitamins may appear when the general nutritional status of the population improves and we begin to see a more limited type of deficiency.

The following generalizations may be made:

(a) The most extensive vitamin deficiency is that of riboflavine, due in part to its very poor absorption from vegetable sources.

(b) Vitamin A deficiency is another very common problem in many parts of the world. In countries where the calorie intake is low, relatively small amounts of fat are consumed. Hence there is a deficiency of fat soluble vitamins. Also the provitamin, β–carotene, is not well absorbed from vegetables. Vitamin A deficiency appears to be a major problem in those countries where there is a prolonged dry season. On the other hand it is interesting to note that in certain parts of West Africa where palm oil is produced, hypervitaminosis A is reported to be occurring.

(c) It is very difficult to generalize about the vitamin C situation for this varies from one area to another. In those regions (usually situated close to the equator) which have a rainfall distributed fairy regularly throughout the year fresh vegetables and fruits are always available. Thus the need for storage of these foods is reduced to a minimum and scurvy is rare. In the regions with a prolonged dry season scurvy is seen not infrequently, and when crop failure also occurs it may be severe.

(d) Although on occasion a pure deficiency of one member of the B group can be found it is usual to find a variable mixed deficiency involving, in addition to riboflavine, thiamine, nicotinic acid, folic acid and occasionally pantothenic acid.

Deficiency of thiamine is still seen in the rice and wheat consuming countries and nicotinamide deficiency where maize is the stable basis of the calories. This problem, in fact, becomes more severe as the country develops economically. Hammer milling of the grain is substituted for the traditional techniques with resulting higher extraction flours and reduced levels of the B group vitamins.

One of the main sources of vitamin B in the past has been locally brewed beer in which the sprouted grain is retained in the final 'brew'. The efforts being made to reduce this local brewing and the substitution of European type beers in urban areas has led to a reduced intake of the B complex.

Virtually nothing is known about the available pyridoxine in these areas. The requirements are probably lower due to the protein deficiency.

(e) A recent survey in East Africa has shown a tocopherol deficiency, but the medical significance of this is not clear.

RELIEF MEASURES

The problem requiring the most urgent solution is how to provide an adequate calorie and protein intake in these countries. Several international groups including the United Nations Children's Fund, the Agency for International Development and the World Health Organization are giving urgent consideration to this problem.

Institutions of food science have been established in many countries and money and technical assistance have been made available for the production of low cost protein-rich food. To date this effort has been concentrated on 'milk' formulae based on locally produced flour (soya bean, cotton seed, maize) with added minerals and in some cases vitamins.

Technical developments are taking place in farming and these measures will lead to steady improvement of the calorie and protein situation. However unless special measures are taken to supplement the diet these present methods could accentuate the vitamin problem as the communities become more urbanized. Adequate surveys of vitamin nutritional status using modern methods are an urgent need in these developing countries in order to ensure appropriate preventive measures.

Part two

The Individual Vitamins

Vitamin A

Retinol

CH₂OH

In 1909 Hopkins and Stepp found that certain fat-soluble substances were necessary for the growth of mice and rats. A fat-soluble growth factor was subsequently extracted from butter and egg yolk by McCollum and Davis (1913–1914). This was designated Vitamine A (the 'e' was later omitted). Its chemical structure was defined by Karrer in 1931, and it was synthesized by Isler (1946–1947). Although vitamin A can be extracted from natural sources, the synthetic vitamin is now used almost exclusively.

CHEMISTRY

Vitamin A is a fat soluble, long chain alcohol which exists in a number of isometric forms. The most active, and that most usually found in mammalian tissues is the all trans vitamin A, which has the structure shown on the previous page. The alcohol is known as retinol and forms pale yellow crystals soluble in fat and fat solvents but not in water. Naturally occuring vitamin A is found only in the animal organism although provitamins (see below) occur in the vegetable kingdom. It is often found in an esterified form and, esters such as the acetate and palmitate are sometimes preferred for nutritional and medicinal use. Vitamin A, especially the free alcohol, is sensitive to oxygen, acids and ultraviolet light. Vitamin A_2 is closely related to vitamin A, but contains an additional double bond in the β-ionone ring. It occurs with vitamin A in fish liver oil.

SOURCES

Vitamin A is only found in the animal kingdom, and a proportion of the daily requirements come from animal sources.

Vitamin A precursors (provitamins) are widely distributed in the vegetable kingdom. These are the carotenoids which have certain structural characteristics and form part of the yellow and orange pigment of most fruit and vegetables:– they include β, β, γ–carotene, β–Apo 8' carotenal and cryptoxanthine.

The main sources of vitamin A and carotene are shown in Table 6. The

Table 6 Content of retinol and β–carotene in certain foods.

	Retinol mg/100 g	β–carotene mg/100 g	Retinol equivalent of β–carotene μg/100 g
Fish liver	up to 300	—	—
Cattle liver	15–150	—	—
Eggs	0·3–0·6	—	—
Milk	up to 0·1	0·03–0.2	5–30
Carrots	—	12·0	2,000
Green beans	—	0·5	80
Margarine (fortified)	1·0	—	—
Butter	0·5–2·0	0·2–1·0	30–170

main dietary intake comes from dairy produce and margarine, which is supplemented with vitamin A in most countries. (page 189)

Since 1969 the content of food and the daily requirement has been based on 'μg retinol equivalent', i.e. retinol is expressed by weight and the carotenoids by the weight of retinol to which they would be converted in the body. Thus:

1 retinol equivalent $= 1$ μg retinol

$= 6$ μg β–carotene

$= 12$ μg other provitamin A carotenoids

$= 3.33$ i.u. vitamin A activity from retinol

$= 10$ i.u. vitamin A activity from β–carotene

Higher daily requirements are now suggested by recent observations.

Although vitamin A is mainly present in the all trans form, other cis-trans isomers can arise in part by spontaneous rearrangement. They are therefore present in varying proportions in different vitamin A preparations.

REQUIREMENTS

The daily requirements for vitamin A in humans are shown on Table 7. These are recommended values and acceptable minimum and optimal values are still based on inadequate evidence. Lower values are acceptable if all is provided as preformed vitamin A, more if all is obtained in the form

Table 7 Daily requirements for vitamin A in humans expressed in μg retinol equivalent/day.

		vitamin A
Adults		μg/day*
Man	Sedentary	1,000
	Moderately active	1,000
	Very active	1,000
Woman	Sedentary	800
	Moderately active	800
	Very active	800
	Pregnancy	1,000
	Lactation	1,200
Children		
Both sexes	Under 1 year	400
	1–3 years	400
	4–6 years	500
	7–9 years	700
	10–12 years	800
Boys	13–15 years	1,000
	16–20 years	1,000
Girls	13–15 years	800
	16–20 years	800

*Expressed as equivalent vitamin A: about one-quarter taken as carotene. If all is taken as vitamin A less is needed.

of carotene. The equivalent values for various animal species are given in Table 36 (page 194). Recent evidence suggests that these requirements may be inadequate but further confirmation is desirable before higher levels are advised.

METABOLISM

The absorption, storage and transport of vitamin A are illustrated in Figure 7. The carotenoids present in the diet can be transformed within the intestinal wall into vitamin A. Of these carotenoids β–carotene is the most useful provitamin. If the β–carotene molecule could be split at the central double bond, then the two molecules of vitamin A would result. In fact the maximum efficiency of conversion appears to be about 50 per cent and the mechanism is probably one of terminal oxidation.

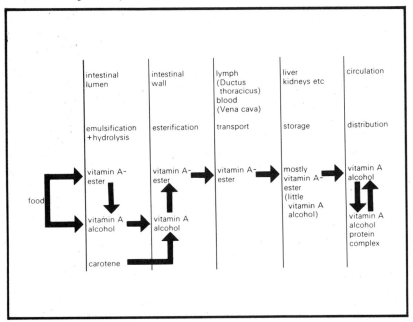

Figure 7 Schematic representation of absorption, storage and transport of vitamin A.

There is active absorption of vitamin A split from the ester form, probably in association with a low density lipoprotein. Absorption is accelerated in the presence of emulsifying agents, e.g. bile. The rate of absorption of vitamin A has been used as a measure of fat absorption. The vitamin is deposited in the Kupffer cells of the liver in an esterified form with long chain fatty acids, mainly retinyl palmitate. It is subsequently carried in the blood bound to a prealbumen-retinol binding protein complex. Recent work suggests that signs of vitamin A deficiency in malnutrition may be due partly to depleted levels of the prealbumen-retinol binding protein transport complex.

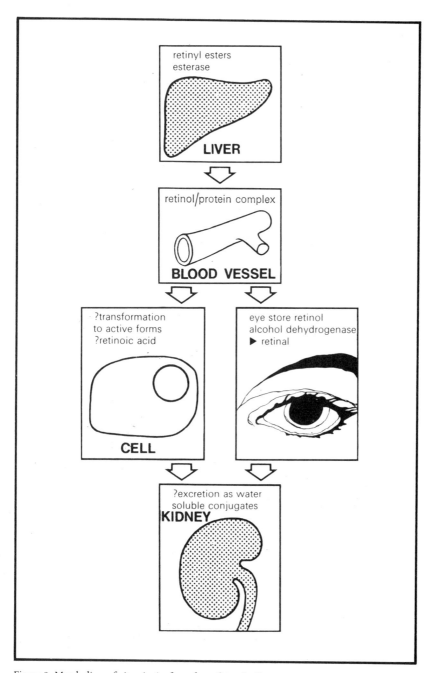

Figure 8 Metabolism of vitamin A after release from the liver.

The further metabolism of vitamin A alcohol released from the liver is shown in Figure 8. Vitamin A is concerned with metabolic integrity within epithelial tissues and in the retina. Recent work shows that some of the peripheral effects can be demonstrated equally well with vitamin A acid, but that this substance can exert only part of the activity within the retina. Vitamin A acid cannot be converted into the alcohol for storage. The acid may be an intermediate or the active compound in these peripheral effects (see below).

PHYSIOLOGY

Vitamin A has an influence on metabolic processes within many cells and a specific role in rod vision.

The mode of action of vitamin A peripherally is still unknown. Its only known actions are in the synthesis of mucopolysaccharides via 'active' sulphate and in the synthesis of corticosterone. It appears to influence the membrane stability of mitochondria and lysosomes. The relative significance of these reactions in the development of the deficiency signs is not clear.

The oxidation of vitamin A alcohol to retinaldehyde is a reversible one, but a further irreversible oxidation to retinoic acid can occur.

Vitamin A alcohol and aldehyde are both capable of maintaining normal vision. Retinoic acid can substitute for either of these substances for normal

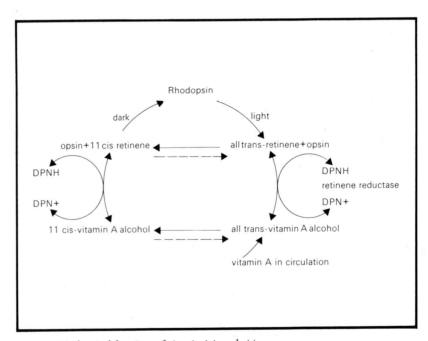

Figure 9 Biochemical functions of vitamin A in rod vision.

44

growth and in some species can maintain normal retinal structure (but not vision). In rodents where such substitution has been undertaken, however, development of the testes is retarded and placental failure occurs in the second half of gestation. In poultry embryo development becomes very abnormal after forty-eight hours and the embryos die.

The visual and reproductive functions are specific to retinol. It is still not certain whether retinoic acid is the natural mediator of some of the other vitamin A effects. Vitamin A plays an integral part in light perception by the rods (Figure 9). The rods of all vertebrates contain a visual pigment with a common chemical structure. This pigment consists of a specific type of protein, opsin, with the 11-cis isomer of vitamin A aldehyde (retinaldehyde, retinene) as chromophore.

The action of light is to change the 11-cis configuration to the all trans form of the retinaldehyde. The further reactions, which produce the sensation of light, are consequences of this but can occur in the dark.

The all trans retinaldehyde cannot form a stable complex with the opsin. The opsin opens through a series of changes exposing reactive groups (Figure 10). Finally the retinaldehyde is hydrolysed off the opsin. Visual excitation occurs during the earlier stages of these reactions.

In vertebrates the all trans retinaldehyde is probably reduced to the vitamin A alcohol and subsequently reoxidised and isomerised to the active 11-cis retinaldehyde. It is however possible that direct isomerisation of released all trans retinaldehyde may occur.

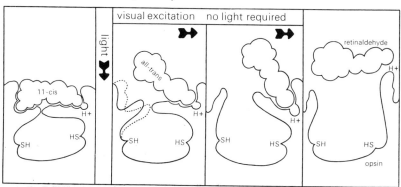

Figure 10 Possible mechanism of rod vision (after Wald).

DEFICIENCY OF VITAMIN A IN ANIMALS

The effect of vitamin A deficiency varies from one animal species to another. The main deficiency disorders are shown in Table 8. The lesions in any species vary according to age, sex and environmental conditions. They are often further complicated by secondary infections and other factors. The pathology reported in the literature is probably not exhaustive for any species, for most authors have concentrated on one effect.

Table 8 Main vitamin A deficiency disorders in animals.

System	Effect
General	Loss of appetite
	Inhibited growth
	Increased susceptibility to infections
	Death
Skin	Dry and scaly
	Poor hair production
Eyes	Night blindness
	Xerophthalmia
	Keratomalacia
Respiratory tract	Extensive keratinisation of lining cells
	Loss of ciliary epithelium
	Multiple infections
Digestive tract	Keratinisation of mucuous membrane
	Loss of gland activities
	Poor absorption
	Infections
Urinary tract	Metaplasia of epithelium and increased tendency to stone formation
Bones	In dogs, overgrowth of porous bone tissue with resulting nerve compression
Male reproductive system	Degeneration of germinal epithelium
Female reproductive system	In fowls—severe degeneration of ovary with decline in egg production and fertility. Infection of genital tract
Foetus	Multiple foetal abnormalities

In common with the majority of vitamin deficiencies, there are signs of a general metabolic defect which manifests itself as retarded growth in young animals or loss of condition and death in mature animals. The main peripheral effect of vitamin A deficiency in most animals is a loss of epithelial integrity with poor resistance to infection (Plate 1). Xerophthalmia is also seen.

The bones show a characteristic overgrowth and nerve lesions may result.

These signs of vitamin A deficiency are still encountered in veterinary practice.

DEFICIENCY OF VITAMIN A IN HUMANS

The main mechanisms by which hypovitaminosis A may develop are shown in Figure 11. In practice vitamin A deficiency and general malnutrition often occur together. Part of the vitamin A deficiency may then be due to poor transport or a result of depleted carrier protein.

The eye

The only unequivocal signs of vitamin A deficiency occur in the eye. These

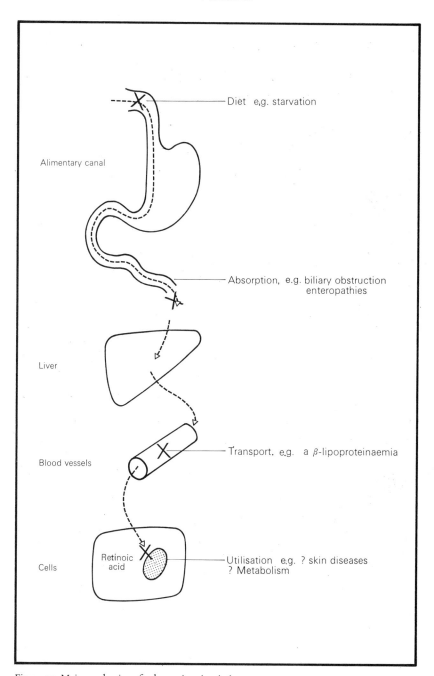

Diet e.g. starvation

Alimentary canal

Absorption, e.g. biliary obstruction
enteropathies

Liver

Transport, e.g. a β-lipoproteinaemia

Blood vessels

Retinoic
acid

Utilisation e.g. ? skin diseases
? Metabolism

Cells

Figure 11 Main mechanisms for hypovitaminosis A.

can be divided into effects on the retina and effects on the anterior segment.

1 *Effect on the retina*
Poor dark adaption is the most constant sign of avitaminosis A. Its incidence can be correlated with the blood level of retinol and it responds rapidly to therapy.

2 *Effect on the anterior segment*
Xerophthalmia, a drying and degenerative disease of the cornea, shows various stages of severity depending on age and other environmental factors. Two stages can be separated:

(a) Xerosis (Plate 3)
Dryness of the conjunctiva with, in children, a wrinkled thickened appearance. Bitot's spots (Plate 4) are often associated with this condition, but their significance may be questioned, for they are also found with normal blood vitamin A levels and rarely respond to vitamin A therapy. The xerosis may extend to the cornea.

(b) Keratomalacia (Plate 5).
At this stage softening of the cornea has occurred. This may be discrete or general and inevitably leads to iris and lens involvement, particularly since secondary infection commonly occurs. Some scarring nearly always remains after therapy. Without treatment total blindness is the usual end result.

The skin
Although skin keratinisation (toad skin) was formerly attributed to vitamin A deficiency it now appears doubtful whether this vitamin is involved and an essential fatty acid deficiency appears more likely.

THERAPY

Deficiency states
Deficiency states should be treated as soon as they occur with high doses of vitamin A, at a daily dose of 20,000–50,000 i.u. daily. Minor grades of vitamin A deficiency can occur with poor absorption (e.g. coeliac disease, gastrectomy), altered metabolism (fever) or excess loss (nephritis). These should be treated with daily doses from 5,000–30,000 units daily. The recent studies are of interest in which single yearly or six monthly oral doses of 300,000 i.u. oil miscible retinol are given as prophylaxis in areas where hypovitaminosis A is endemic.

Other disorders
The only established signs of vitamin A deficiency in the human are the eye lesions and such patients should be treated as above. In addition vitamin A

therapy is given extensively in a wide range of diseases including dermatoses, acne, senile vaginitis, atrophic rhinitis and anosmia. A daily dose of 50,000 units is usually given. For certain skin disorders (e.g. psoriasis, certain ichthyoses, acne vulgaris) topical retinoic acid appears to be effective therapy.

HYPERVITAMINOSIS

There have been isolated reports of hypervitaminosis A occuring in children after prolonged high dosage. Skin changes (dry rough skin), hepatomegaly and painful joint swellings are seen, but they disappear on withholding the vitamin.

Vitamin D

Calciferol

The first description of rickets was given by Whistler in 1645. Its association with lack of sunlight was suggested by Palm in 1890 and in 1919 cure by ultraviolet light was discussed for the first time. The isolation of the active sterols from natural sources and from irradiated provitamins was undertaken during the 1930s. In 1969 it was discovered that the vitamin is metabolized to a calcium controlling hormone.

CHEMISTRY

Vitamin D is present in nature in several forms. All are sterols and occur only in the animal organism. Vitamin D_3 (cholecalciferol) derived from 7-dehydrocholesterol by ultraviolet irradiation occurs in human skin and is found in liver oils. The active synthetic compound for therapy in the human is Vitamin D_2 (ergocalciferol). It occurs as colourless crystals, insoluble in water but readily soluble in alcohol and other organic solvents. It is less soluble in vegetable oils.

SOURCES

The active form of vitamin D is not widely distributed in nature, although provitamins D are present in many vegetables. The only rich sources are the liver and viscera of fish (vitamin D_3). The average contents are given in Table 9. Certain foods, including milk, can have their content increased by irradiation. Vitamin D supplements are included in margarine.

Table 9 Content of vitamin D (as D_3) in certain foods.

	Vitamin D_3 i.u./100 g
Milk	2
Cheese	10
Eggs	50–170[*]
Meat	4
Sea Fish (fatty types) – oils	0–50,000
Butter	40
Margarine (fortified)	300

[*] If poultry are fed vitamin D supplement

Recent studies have shown that in most climatic conditions, normal adults obtain adequate amounts of vitamin D by exposure to sunlight. The need for dietary vitamin is only apparent under special conditions, particularly in sunless climates. In Great Britain seasonal variation of vitamin D levels are found and most people need some vitamin D in their diet.

REQUIREMENTS

The normal human requirement is still unknown. A daily dietary requirement of 400 i.u. (10 μg cholecalciferol) has been suggested for women dur-

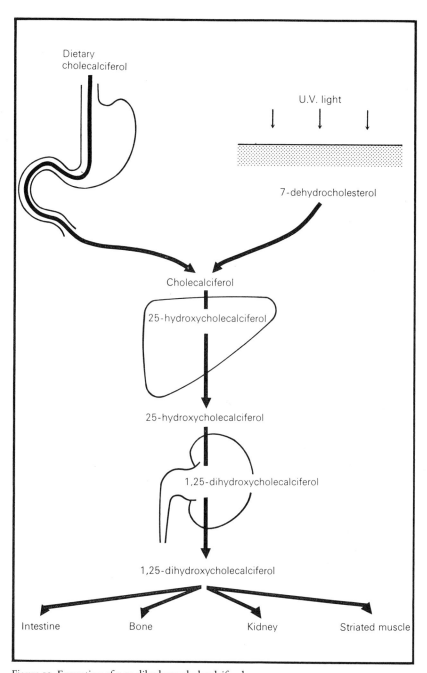

Figure 12 Formation of 1,25-dihydroxycholecalciferol.

ing pregnancy and lactation; for children and for the elderly. For normal adults whose exposure to sunlight may be inadequate, daily intake up to 400 i.u. is justified. The optimum levels for various animal species are shown in Table 36 (page 194).

METABOLISM
Vitamin D is absorbed from the intestinal tract in association with fats, as are all the fat soluble vitamins. Like the rest, it needs the presence of bile salts for absorption.

Of greater interest than the absorption of the dietary vitamin is the biogenesis of the vitamin. Cholecalciferol (vitamin D_3) is formed in the skin by the action of ultraviolet light on the precursor 7-dehydrocholesterol (Figure 12).

Cholecalciferol (or synthetic ergocalciferol) is converted to 25-hydroxy-cholecalciferol in the liver and then further hydroxylated in the kidney to 1,25-dihydroxycholecalciferol – the active hormone form. The formation of the 1,25-dihydroxy form in the kidney is under the control of parathyroid hormone probably through the intermediary of kidney parenchyma phosphate levels (Figure 12).

The formation and high concentration of vitamin D in the fish liver has not yet been explained.

PHYSIOLOGY
Vitamin D is intimately concerned with the metabolism of calcium and phosphorus. The principal action of the vitamin is to increase the absorption of calcium and phosphorus from the intestine. It also has a direct effect on the calcification process by increasing the uptake of minerals by bone. Within the kidney vitamin D increases the clearance of phosphate.

In addition to these effects on calcium and phosphorus, vitamin D increases tissue citrate levels and, consequently, increases citrate excretion.

These effects are brought about by alterations in the level of calcium binding proteins (at least two with different molecular weights are known) under the control of the hormone 1,25-dihydroxycholecalciferol.

DEFICIENCY OF VITAMIN D IN ANIMALS
Symptoms and signs of vitamin D deficiency are seen mainly in young animals. General consequences of a deficiency can appear in the form of an inhibition of growth and a loss of weight, reduced or lost appetite, accelerated respiration (in the calf) and also increased sensitivity and incidence of cramp (tetany—especially in young pigs) before the characteristic signs which relate primarily to the bone system, become apparent. These latter take the form of enlargement of the epiphyses, curvature and increased brittleness of the bones in the extremities (Figure 13), sternum, vertebral column, pelvis and cranium. Formation of the teeth and dentition are also disturbed. The animals move stiffly and hesitantly, they have defective posture, lameness and muscular weakness, or they lie still.

In poultry, a deficiency of vitamin D is manifested also in the production of eggs with thin shells; production of eggs falls and their fertility is considerably impaired. The beaks of rachitic chickens are soft and pliant.

In cattle and sheep severe vitamin D deficiency during gestation leads to the birth of weak, dead or deformed young.

Although now rare with good animal husbandry, rickets is still encountered in veterinary practice.

DEFICIENCY OF VITAMIN D IN HUMANS

Deficiency of vitamin D during childhood leads to the development of rickets. In adults, deficiency causes osteomalacia. The features which differentiate rickets

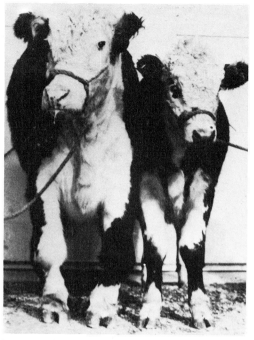

Figure 13 Cow on left developed rickets early in life when maintained on a vitamin D deficient diet with no direct sunlight. Note bowed legs and large joints. By courtesy of Dr. L. L. Madsen, Utah State Agr. College, Logan, Utah.

from osteomalacia are due to the fact that the ends of the bones of children are in a state of active growth. This growth is modified by rickets in such a way as to give rise to enlargements and deformities which are never seen in osteomalacia because in the adult person the epiphyseal cartilage does not exist. The overriding abnormality is in calcium metabolism and the causes of reduced body calcium are shown in Table 10. This tentative classification of osteodystrophies due to hypocalcaemia is based upon our new idea of the pathophysiology.

Rickets

Usually the first symptoms of rickets to attract attention are excessive sweating and gastrointestinal disturbances. In reality, however, the earliest signs are the deformities of the skeleton, of which the first to appear is craniotabes, this sometimes being seen as early as the second month. Craniotabes consists of areas of softening of the skull, almost always located in the occipital and parietal bones along the lambdoidal sutures. Later there may be thickening of the cranial vault giving rachitic 'bossing of the skull' (Figure 14). Primary dentition may be delayed and the disease often causes the teeth

Table 10 Clinical presentation of hypocalcaemic osteodystrophies.

Disorders	Pathophysiology
	(1) Dietary deficiency:
Infantile rickets; osteomalacia	(a) of vitamin D
High diet phytic acid, fats, etc.	(b) calcium binding
	(2) Deficient absorption:
Biliary obstruction	(a) bile salt deficiency
Coeliac disease ? Post gastrectomy	(b) intestinal defect
Primary biliary cirrhosis	(3) Liver abnormalities
Anticonvulsant therapy	
Chronic renal insufficiency	(4) Renal abnormalities:
Cushing's disease	(a) renal cell defect
Glucocorticoid therapy	(b) ? inhibition of 1α-hydroxylase
Strontium poisoning	
? Some familial resistant rickets	(c) absent 1α-hydroxylase
Familial hypophosphataemia	(d) hypophosphataemia
Wilson's disease	
Cystinosis	
Fanconi syndrome	
Hypoparathyroidism	(5) No parathyroid feed-back
? Certain malabsorption types	(6) Reduced intestinal sensitivity to 1,25-DHCC
Resistant rickets	

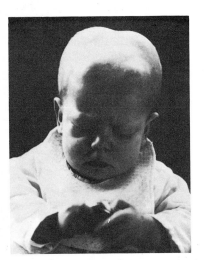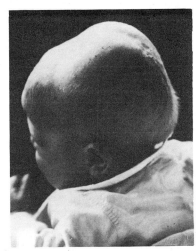

Figure 14 Vitamin D deficiency in male twins of 16 months showing typical 'skull bossing'.

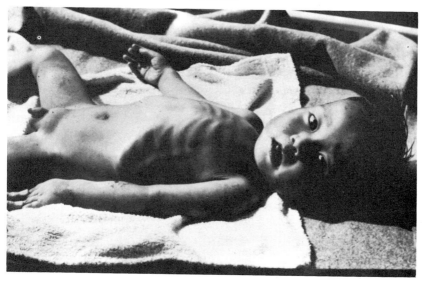

Figure 15 Rickety rosary in a young child. Reproduced from 'Assessment of Nutritional Status of a Community' by D. B. Jelliffe (1966) by permission of the World Health Organization.

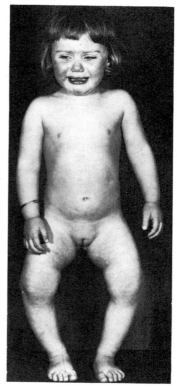

Figure 16 Pronounced bowing of the tibia in a rachitic child of 2 years. By courtesy of Dr. P. Hansell, Westminster Hospital, London S.W.1.

to erupt out of order. After craniotabes, the next sign to appear is enlargement of the costochondral junctions giving the 'rachitic rosary' (Figure 15). The spine becomes deformed posturally but not in actual structure. Rickets produces enlargements of the ends of long bones and the shafts of these bones may be curved in various directions, depending on the age at which rickets developed. Thus, after the second year 'bow' legs are common (Figure 16). When the child with severe rickets begins to walk, the gait has a characteristic waddling appearance. Pelvic bone deformation due to rickets is an important cause of dystocia in adult women. Rickets also affects the muscles resulting in 'pot-belly' appearance. Stunting of growth may be extreme.

Osteomalacia

Vitamin D deficiency arising in adults leads to osteomalacia. The reactions of the skeleton in rickets and osteomalacia are fundamentally similar. However, while there are unfused epiphyses in the child, these are fused by adult life. The different clinical signs arise from this.

In osteomalacia there is gradually increasing rarefaction of the bones. Those of the pelvis, thorax and extremities are particularly involved. The pelvis shows characteristic deformation. The sacrum convexity is increased, the rims of the iliac bone are flattened, the inlet becomes asymmetrical and narrowed. Normal parturition is almost impossible in osteomalacia.

In the bones of the extremities, the cortex becomes thin. Spontaneous fractures occur.

Senile osteoporosis

Most elderly patients show some degree of bone rarefaction and fractures after minor trauma are common. An inadequate level of cholecalciferol is a factor in its genesis.

Vitamin D resistant rickets

Numerous syndromes have been described in which bone rarefaction resistant to heroic doses of vitamin D is a feature. These have been grouped under the broad term of 'vitamin D resistant rickets'. Our new ideas about the metabolism of cholecalciferol into the hormone 1,25-dehydroxycholecalciferol suggest a more rational approach to the classification of their geneses. A tentative classification is given in Table 10.

THERAPY

Deficiency states

The principal use of vitamin D is in the prophylaxis and treatment of disorders of calcium-phosphorus metabolism. In infants and younger children rickets, spasmophilia and tetany are often due to a low blood calcium. The prevention and treatment of rickets require an adequate dietary intake of calcium, phosphorus and vitamin D. The need for the vitamin is considerably increased during pregnancy and lactation. Senile osteoporosis may be due to lack of vitamin D and therefore all elderly persons should receive adequate amounts.

The prophylactic dose is 1,000 to 4,000 units daily. For therapy doses up to 20,000 units daily may be given.

Other disorders

With our greater understanding of the genesis of 'vitamin D resistant rickets' have come advances in therapy. Successful trials in renal rickets and related disorders have been carried out with minute doses of 1,25-dihydroxycholecalciferol and related compounds. It is still too early to give a final assessment on the most effective compound.

One of the indications for ergocalciferol therapy is long term administration of antiepileptic drugs. It is interesting to note that the administration of ergocalciferol also reduces the incidence of epileptic attacks.

HYPERVITAMINOSIS

Ingestion of massive doses has been shown to cause widespread calcification of soft tissues including lungs and kidneys. It is particularly important to avoid the administration of large doses in infants, whose daily intake should not exceed 400 units.

Extreme sensitivity to vitamin D, such that even normal intake produces hypervitaminosis is seen in sarcoidosis and in hereditary nephrocalcinosis.

Vitamin E

Tocopherol

The effect of vitamin E deficiency was first noted by Matthill and Conklin in 1920 when they found that there were reproduction abnormalities in rats kept on special milk diets. Evans and Bishop (1922) showed that these abnormalities could be prevented by a factor in lettuce and wheat germ oil. This factor was isolated in 1936 by Evans and his group and total synthesis achieved in 1938 (Karrer *et al.*). Vitamin E was recognized as essential for human nutrition by the Food and Nutrition Board of the USA in 1959.

CHEMISTRY

α-Tocopherol, an alcohol derived from phytol and a trimethyl hydroquinone, has the structure shown at the beginning of the chapter. Several related tocopherols have also been isolated from natural sources, but their biological activity is less than the α form. α-Tocopherol is a yellow oil, insoluble in water, soluble in organic solvents. It is readily oxidized. The acetate which shows similar biological activity is more stable.

SOURCES

Tocopherols are present in small quantities in many plants, including lettuce, grasses, peanuts and the embryos of many seeds. They are also found in milk and milk products and egg yolks.

It must be borne in mind that α-tocopherol is the most effective vitamin E, but that other tocopherols are also present in varying proportions.

Seed oils contain the highest levels, up to about 50 mg α-tocopherol per 100 ml.

REQUIREMENTS

In humans natural deficiency is only seen as a result of absorption defect disorders but from experimental studies it can be concluded that a daily intake of between 3 and 15 mg of tocopherol is required on a normal diet. Amounts in excess of 15 mg are probably needed when large amounts of unsaturated fatty acids are included in the diet. The daily requirement in infants is 5–10 mg. For animals the optimum supply is shown in Table 36 (page 194).

METABOLISM

The absorption of vitamin E is similar to that of other fat soluble vitamins in that it is probably linked to fat absorption and facilitated by the presence of bile salts. In normal people about 70 per cent of an ingested dose is absorbed. Vitamin E may itself facilitate the absorption of vitamin A and carotene storage takes place in the liver and there is a linear relationship between tocopherol content of the diet and liver storage. The metabolism of tocopherol is still in doubt and it is still not known whether the parent compound is the active form at cellular level.

In man the normal serum level of tocopherol is about 1·0 mg/100 ml. Newborn infants, however, show a considerably lower value (about 0·2– 0·4 mg/100 ml). High tocopherol levels have been found in the fat, liver, heart. and adrenal cortex. The remaining tissues have levels similar to those of the serum.

PHYSIOLOGY

Vitamin E has a powerful anti-oxidant effect within the animal body, particularly for lipids. It is very closely involved in metabolism with the mineral selenium and the two substances appear to be interdependent in most species. By their joint action a sparing of Vitamin A and of polyunsaturated fatty acids occurs. The antioxidant effect may occur at the mitochondrial membrane. It may be one of the factors that maintain low cellular enzyme toxic peroxide levels. However, antioxidant activity alone does not explain all the experimental data and the full mechanism of action of vitamin E is still unsolved. A role in intracellular respiration is postulated, possibly by an action on ubiquinone and co-enzyme A levels.

Nucleic acid metabolism also appears to be deranged in vitamin E deficiency.

DEFICIENCY OF VITAMIN E IN ANIMALS

Using appropriate diets, pathological evidence of vitamin E deficiency can be produced in most animal species. The most common of these are shown in Table 11 (but vitamin E deficiency has been found in all other species

Table 11 Main reported tocopherol deficiency diseases in animal species.

Lesion	Rat	Rabbit	Dog	Fowl	Sheep	Cattle	Monkey
Testes degeneration	+	+	+	+			
Foetal resorption	+						
Muscle dystrophy	+	+	+	+	+	+	+
Hyaline necrosis	+	+			+	+	+
Ceroid pigmentation	+		+	+			+
Nervous system degeneration	+			+		+	+
Vascular system defects	+	+	+	+		+	+

that have been studied). The main signs of deficiency are degeneration of the testis, abnormalities of gestation, muscular dystrophy (Plate 6) and central nervous system and vascular system defects. Other abnormalities reported include regression in the ovary and decreased egg hatchability.

Muscular dystrophy (e.g. stiff lamb disease), 'mulberry heart disease' of pigs, central nervous system degeneration, e.g. encephalopathy ('crazy chick disease') and foetal resorption due to hypovitaminosis E/selenium deficiency have all been encountered in veterinary practice.

DEFICIENCY OF VITAMIN E IN HUMANS

Deficiency disease in an otherwise normal human has not been reported but the general causes of a deficiency are shown in Figure 17. Some evidence of

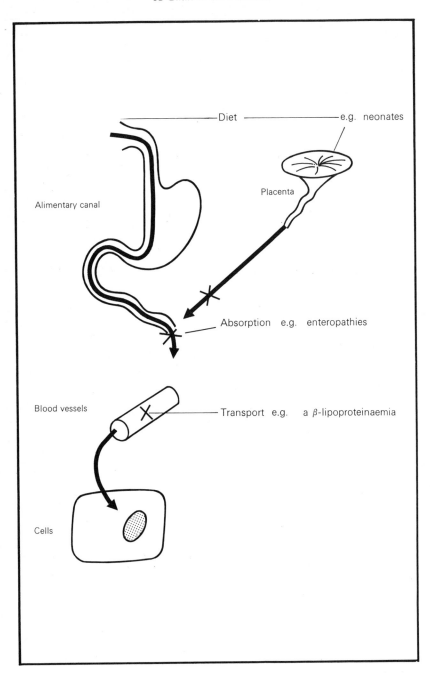

Figure 17 Mechanisms for hypovitaminosis E.

deficiency is seen in children with fat absorption defects (e.g. sprue, fibrocystic disease of the pancreas). Creatinuria, ceroid pigmentation and abnormal red cell haemolysis are encountered. Similar features, possibly associated with inadequate carrier protein, are seen in the rare disorder, hypobeta lipoproteinaemia.

Fat absorption defects in adults also cause biochemical evidence of low tocopherol levels.

Human tocopherol deficiency has been produced by artificial diets high in unsaturated fatty acids. Biochemical evidence of deficiency can be determined and other findings include a diminished erythrocyte lifespan and peptic ulceration. The significance of the latter finding is not certain, but irritation from autoxidised fats appears to be the most likely cause.

Neonates show low tocopherol levels, and it is important to ensure that these are not further aggravated by the use of artificial diets low in tocopherol since premature infants fed on diets low in tocopherol develop a haemolytic anaemia when about 8 weeks old.

THERAPY

Deficiency states
Supplementation is desirable in fat malabsorption syndromes; in premature infants on artificial foods and when large amounts of unsaturated fatty acids are included in the diet. The dosage varies from 10 mg daily in infants to about 30 mg in older children and adults.

Other disorders
Vitamin E has been used extensively in clinical medicine but careful examination of the evidence available reveals that in the majority of instances there is inadequate evidence to prove its value. In particular, no effect on human muscular dystrophy has been proved.

There is, however, well founded evidence for the value of large doses of tocopherol (400–600 mg per day over a prolonged period) in intermittent claudication.

In addition there is a reasonable evidence for the administration of tocopherol (up to 400 mg per day) to patients with stasis ulcers and in certain fibrous tissue degenerations (Peyronie's disease, Dupuytren's contracture).

Vitamin K

The general term vitamin K is now used to describe not a single chemical entity, but a group of quinone compounds which have characteristic antihaemorrhagic effects.

The presence of a dietary antihaemorrhagic factor was first suspected in 1929, when haemorrhage was noted in chicks maintained on a low fat diet. Related compounds were isolated from different sources from 1935 to 1939 and the chemical constitution and synthesis accomplished in 1939.

CHEMISTRY

A large number of chemical compounds possess some degree of vitamin K activity. They are all related to 2-methyl-1, 4-naphtho-quinone. The most important vitamin K form which occurs naturally is vitamin K_1 (originally isolated from lucerne). It is soluble only in organic solvents. Many related active compounds have been synthesized. Some of these have the advantage of being water soluble. Among the most widely used of these is the tetra-sodium salt of 2-methyl-1,4-naphtho-hydroquinone diphosphate ('Synkavit'). This compound occurs as colourless water soluble crystals, stable in solution.

SOURCES

Vitamin K_1 is distributed fairly widely in nature. The main sources are shown in Table 12 from which it can be seen that vitamin K is only found in abundance in brassica and in spinach. In addition to these sources, however, many bacteria including some of the normal intestinal flora can synthesize vitamin K.

REQUIREMENTS

Vitamin K is synthesized in the intestine and this endogenous material is probably absorbed. Hence no accurate estimate can be made of the daily

Table 12 Content of vitamin K in certain foods.

	Vitamin K mg/100 g
Lean meat	0·1–0·2
Ox liver	0·1–0·2
Pig liver	0·4–0·8
Eggs (each)	0·02
Cow's milk	0·002
Human milk	0·02
Potatoes	0·08
Spinach	0·6
Green cabbage	0·4
Carrots	0·01
Peas	0·01–0·03
Tomatoes	0·4

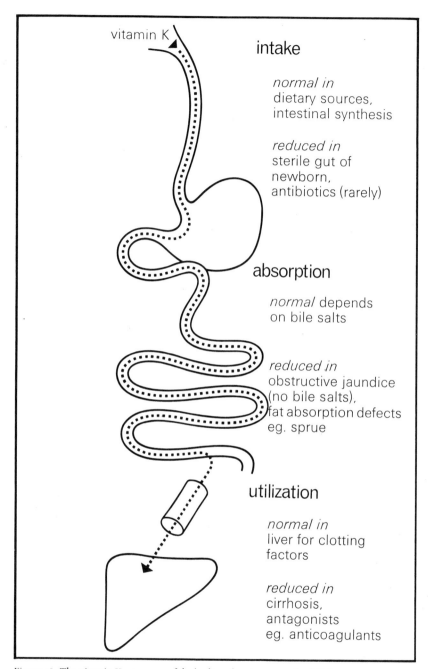

vitamin K

intake

normal in
dietary sources,
intestinal synthesis

reduced in
sterile gut of
newborn,
antibiotics (rarely)

absorption

normal depends
on bile salts

reduced in
obstructive jaundice
(no bile salts),
fat absorption defects
eg. sprue

utilization

normal in
liver for clotting
factors

reduced in
cirrhosis,
antagonists
eg. anticoagulants

Figure 18 The vitamin K economy of the body and main causes of a deficiency.

requirements of the normal adult, but from animal experiments and experience in the newborn, they are probably between 20 and 100 μg in adults and less than 10 μg in infants. The intake and production within the body is normally more than adequate. In babies during the first day or so of life at which time they have not developed an intestinal flora a daily intake of about 1 mg daily is required.

Estimated requirements for animals are shown on Table 36 (page 194).

METABOLISM

Vitamin K, like all the oil soluble vitamins, is absorbed in association with the dietary fats and requires the presence of bile salts for adequate uptake from the alimentary canal (Figure 18). After the absorption the vitamin is utilized in the liver. Very little is stored and the rest is metabolized. The poor storage means that rapid depletion occurs, probably within about a week, if absorption is reduced.

Several antagonists to vitamin K are now known. These include related quinones (e.g. 2-chloro-3-phytyl-1,4-naphthaquinone), coumarin derivatives and indanediones. These two latter groups of compounds are used as anticoagulants.

PHYSIOLOGY

The most important physiological function for vitamin K is the production of certain co-agulation factors in the blood plasma. These factors are proteins produced in the liver and their synthesis depends on the presence of minute quantities of vitamin K. This probably acts on the incorporation of sugars in proteins at a post-ribosomal stage. The clotting factors which it is at present believed are K-dependent are: Prothrombin; Proconvertin – Factor VII; Christmas Factor – Factor IX; Stuart-Prower Factor – Factor X.

DEFICIENCY OF VITAMIN K IN ANIMALS

Haemorrhagic disease due to vitamin K deficiency can be produced experimentally in

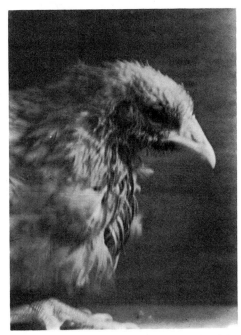

Figure 19 Typical appearance of vitamin K deficiency in a young chick. Note ruffled feathers and bloody discharge.

many animals, either by dietary restriction in some species (chicks) or by feeding antagonists. To produce a deficiency which is severe enough to cause symptoms it is usually necessary to destroy the intestinal flora with antibiotics. Natural vitamin K deficiency haemorrhagic states in mammals are rare, but calves and piglets can occasionally develop bleeding at mucous membranes or into organs; this can be cured or prevented by vitamin K.

Vitamin K deficiency has greater practical significance in the case of poultry, especially in the young. It is manifested in slight cases by general weakness, rough plumage (Figure 19) paleness and icteric colouration of the comb, wattles and eye-lids as a result of anaemia. Characteristic signs of pronounced deficiency of vitamin K are subcutaneous and intramuscular haemorrhages which lead to bluish-red colourations in different parts of the body. Blood appears in the faeces and, on dissection, bleeding is to be found in the crop and appendix. Haemorrhages occur in mucous membranes and organs.

The most common cause of vitamin K deficiency in veterinary practice is the accidental poisoning of domestic animals with warfarin sodium. This is used as a rodenticide and depletes prothrombin (page 70). Domestic animals suffering from warfarin poisoning should be treated with vitamin K_1.

DEFICIENCY OF VITAMIN K IN HUMANS
The mode of production of haemorrhagic diseases due to avitaminosis K is shown in Figure 18. It may be caused by:

1 Inadequate intake and production causing haemorrhagic disease of the newborn (Plate 8).

A decrease in the prothrombin level normally occurs in infants shortly after birth, when the supply from the maternal blood begins to diminish and the intestinal flora of the infant is not yet sufficiently established to produce vitamin K. Milk is a very poor source of vitamin K.

Even small haemorrhages occurring in vital structures (e.g. brain) can be so serious that it is now established practice to give a small dose of vitamin K prophylactically immediately after birth to all infants.

2 Deficient absorption as in sprue or obstructive jaundice. A common problem is haemorrhage at operation for obstructive jaundice. For this reason any patient being operated on for obstructive jaundice should receive vitamin K therapy beforehand. The preferred treatment is phylloquinone parenterally.

3 Induced by anticoagulant therapy.

Oral 'prothrombin' reducing agents of the coumarin or indanedione type are now established for anticoagulant therapy. They act as vitamin K antagonists. During anticoagulant therapy dangerously low prothrombin levels can be corrected rapidly and effectively by the administration of vitamin K_1 but it does *not* respond to the water soluble synthetic analogues.

4 Inadequate utilization.

Low prothrombin levels are frequently encountered in patients with various liver disorders including viral hepatitis, cirrhosis and malignant disease of the liver and only rarely respond to vitamin K administration.

THERAPY

Deficiency state

As an antidote to anticoagulant therapy vitamin K_1 is the only effective compound. For other conditions in which poor absorption is the primary defect one of the synthetic analogues may be substituted for the natural vitamin K_1.

1 In the neonatal period. Prophylactically or therapeutically for haemorrhagic disease of the newborn. Vitamin K_1 intramuscularly $0 \cdot 5$–$1 \cdot 0$ mg.

2 Doses for haemorrhagic disease associated with poor absorption or inadequate utilization. Synthetic analogues (e.g. 'Synkavit') 10–40 mg by mouth daily or Vitamin K_1 1–5 mg intramuscularly.

3 Antidote to anticoagulant therapy.

Synthetic analogues (e.g. 'Synkavit') have no place as antidotes in anticoagulant therapy.

(a) Haemorrhage. Vitamin K_1 10 mg intramuscularly or by slow intravenous injection. The prothrombin level should be estimated again three hours later and a further dose given if necessary.

(b) Lowering of prothrombin to potentially dangerous levels. Vitamin K_1 5–10 mg by mouth. High doses should be avoided if it is intended to continue with anticoagulant therapy.

Other disorders

Certain synthetic vitamin K analogues, particularly 'Synkavit', have been shown to act as radiosensitizing agents. Doses of 50–100 mg are administered by intravenous injection just before each X-ray treatment.

Thiamine

Vitamin B$_1$ Aneurine

The disease beri-beri was recognized in China as early as 2600 B.C. and is probably the earliest documented deficiency disorder. No cure was found until the investigations of Takaki (1884) on the effects of diet. In 1890 Eijkman produced experimental avian polyneuritis, a condition resembling beri-beri, and showed that the curative factor was a water soluble substance present in rice-polishings. In 1901 Grijns first suggested that beri-beri and avian polyneuritis resulted from the lack in the diet of certain substances of importance to the metabolism of the nervous system. The isolation of the active component occurred during the 1910s, but the determination of the constitution and the first synthesis did not take place until the mid 1930s.

CHEMISTRY

The thiamine molecule consists of a pyrimidine ring and a thiazole component linked by a methylene bridge. It contains a quarternary N atom. It is a water soluble, white crystalline solid. It is oxidized by potassium ferricyanide in the presence of alkali to thiochrome. The stability of thiamine is good, even in heat, if it is in the crystallized state or in an acid solution. In a neutral or alkaline solution the stability of thiamine is not good. It is also sensitive to ultraviolet light.

SOURCES

Thiamine is present in high concentration in yeast and in the pericarp and germ of cereals. The main dietary sources of thiamine are shown in Table 13; however, thiamine is present in practically all plant and animal tissues. Widely used cereal products – bread, breakfast cereals etc, are now enriched with thiamine and these sources probably provide as much as 30 to 40 per cent of the daily intake.

REQUIREMENTS

The requirement is increased when carbohydrate is taken in large amounts and reduced when fat and protein provide a large proportion of the daily calories. The requirements are increased during periods of increased metabolism, e.g. fever, hyperthyroidism, muscular activity and also pregnancy and during lactation.

An average requirement of about 0·5 mg per 1,000 kcal has been

Table 13 Content of thiamine in certain foods.

		Thiamine mg/100 g		Thiamine mg/100 g
			Beef	up to 0·6
Wheat flour	Wholemeal	0·36–0·5	Lamb	0·1–0·2
	85% extraction	0·3–0·4	Pork	up to 1·0
	73% ,,	0·07–0·1	Poultry	0·1
			Peas	0·36
Rice	Whole rice	0·5	Other legumes	0·4–0·6
	Polished rice	0·03	Potatoes	0·08–0·1
	Rice bran	2·3	Cows milk	0·045

recommended (equivalent to 1·5 mg/day) with increase in stress conditions. The minimum is estimated at about 1·0 mg/day on an average diet in normal conditions. The recommended daily intake is shown in Table 14.

The optimum daily intake for various animal species is given in Table 36 (page 194).

Table 14 Daily requirements for thiamine in humans expressed in mg/day.

		Thiamine mg/day
Adults		
Man	Sedentary	1·2
	Moderately active	1·6
	Very active	1·8
Women	Sedentary	1·0
	Moderately active	1·2
	Very active	1·4
	Pregnancy	1·4
	Lactation	1·4
Children		
Both sexes	Under 1 year	0·4
	1–3 years	0·7
	4–6 years	0·9
	7–9 years	1·1
	10–12 years	1·3
Boys	13–15 years	1·4
	16–20 years	1·5
Girls	13–15 years	1·2
	16–20 years	1·2

METABOLISM

Thiamine can be synthesized by plants and perhaps in some lower animals. In mammals bacteria in the intestinal tract may synthesize some thiamine. The extent of this synthesis depends on a large number of factors including dietary intake. Mammals are almost completely dependent on dietary thiamine in most circumstances.

Thiamine is rapidly and actively absorbed from the small intestine and within the body is transformed by phosphorylation into active co-enzyme thiamine pyrophosphate (cocarboxylase).

The reaction can take place in most tissues but particularly in the liver cells. The blood level amounts to about 10 μg/100 ml as cocarboxylase in the corpuscles and about 1 μg as the free vitamin in the plasma. Larger quantities of cocarboxylase (up to 0·1 mg/100 ml) may be found in the leucocytes.

Small amounts of the phosphorylated form occur in all animal cells, but the body is incapable of storing the free vitamin. Dephosphorylation can occur in the kidney (and probably in other organs) and excess quantities of the free vitamin and pyrimidine are excreted in the urine. The urinary excretion depends in part on the urine volume and during diuresis large amounts of thiamine may be lost. Small quantities are excreted in the sweat.

In certain fish (e.g. carp) there is a heat labile enzyme (thiaminase) which destroys thiamine. This has led to signs of thiamine deficiency in certain animals (e.g. foxes) to which the raw fish has been fed. In those countries where large amounts of fish are eaten raw, human thiamine deficiency may also occur. Some bacteria (e.g. *Bacillus thiaminolyticus*) are also capable of destroying thiamine. It has been reported that some 3 per cent of Japanese show a thiamine deficiency due to this cause.

Other direct antagonists include oxythiamine and pyrithiamine.

PHYSIOLOGY

Thiamine in the form of thiamine pyrophosphate is:

1 The co-enzyme in certain bacteria for the decarboxylation of α-keto-fatty acids, e.g. pyruvic acid; α-ketoglutaric acid. The typical reaction is:

$$CH_3COCOOH \rightarrow CH_3CHO + CO_2.$$

2 In animals there is oxidative decarboxylation whereby the oxidized form of acetaldehyde (acetic acid) is formed. For this reaction co-enzyme A (page 127), lipoic acid and nicotinamide adenine dinucleotide (NAD) are required in addition to thiamine pyrophosphate. This reaction is shown diagrammatically in Figure 20, but probably involves many stages.

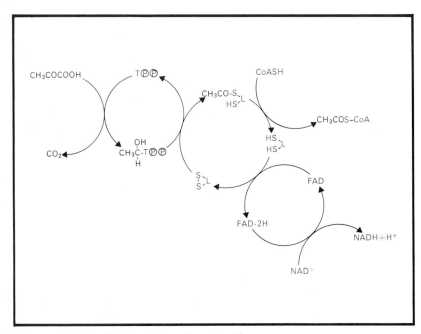

Figure 20 Oxidative decarboxylation of pyruvic acid.

This oxidative decarboxylation is an extremely important reaction in animals, for it yields the two carbon fragment, activated as acetyl-co-enzyme A (Co A), which forms both the link between carbohydrates, fats and proteins and the mode of entry of carbohydrates into the citric acid cycle (page 8).

In the case of α-ketoglutaric acid similar reactions yield succinyl Co A.

3 The co-enzyme for transketolation reactions in the pentose phosphate cycle. Erythrocytes from thiamine deficient animals show an impairment of this cycle with an accumulation of pentoses.

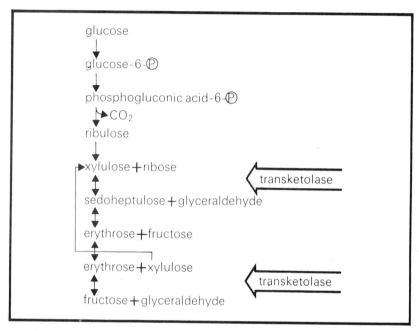

Figure 21 Part played by thiamine-dependent transketolase in the direct oxidative pathway for glucose.

The reactions of the pentose phosphate cycle (sometimes known as the hexose monophosphate shunt) are shown in Figure 21. Its principal functions are:

(a) To provide pentose phosphate for nucleotide synthesis.

(b) To supply reduced NADP for various synthetic pathways, e.g. fatty acid synthesis – steroid hydroxylation. The glycolytic breakdown of glucose forms exclusively reduced NAD.

It is relatively unimportant as a source of energy though the proportion of glucose metabolized by this route is high in the lactating mammary gland, adrenal cortex, leucocytes and erythrocytes.

From these important reactions it will be seen that thiamine is an important factor in carbohydrate metabolism. In thiamine deficiency blood pyruvate, and often blood lactate rises steeply. It is not certain whether the central nervous system effects of thiamine deficiency should be attributed to these effects on carbohydrate metabolism or to the resulting decrease in active acetate components for production of acetylcholine.

DEFICIENCY OF THIAMINE IN ANIMALS

Thiamine deficiency disorders have been described for many animal species. In view of the close relationship between vitamin B_1 and the metabolism of carbohydrates, it is obvious that a deficiency of this vitamin produces disorders in the function of the organs and tissues, where there is much metabolism of carbohydrates. It means that the nervous system and heart are affected, and also the liver, gastrointestinal tract and muscle tissue.

The main effects of thiamine deficiency are shown in Table 15. The

Table 15 Main effects of thiamine deficiency in animals.

System	Effect
General	Loss of appetite
	Weight loss
	General weakness and death
Heart	Fatty degeneration and necrosis of heart fibres
	Bradycardia
	Heart failure
Liver	Fatty degeneration and haemorrhages
Intestinal tract	Mucosal inflammation
	Ulcers and haemorrhages
Central nervous system	Progressive paralysis leading to death
	In birds typical neck retraction occurs
Skin	Skin oedema and cyanosis
Testes	Development inhibited in young cocks
Ovaries	Atrophied
	Reduced egg production and hatchability in hens
Motor end plate	In some species degeneration
Muscle tissue	Diffuse degeneration with fibre swelling and vacuolation

animal grows more slowly or loses weight. In birds and young animals a characteristic neck retraction (Figure 22) results from the nerve paralysis. Modification of the motor end plate has been reported in some species. This nerve paralysis progresses to respiratory failure and death. In the intestinal tract inflammatory changes and ulcers are present. The heart shows very extensive atrophic changes. The animals developing thiamine deficiency most readily are chickens and pigeons: less readily depleted are pigs, rats, mice and rabbits, probably due to endogenous thiamine production.

In ruminants production of thiamine in the intestinal tract renders thiamine deficiency unlikely.

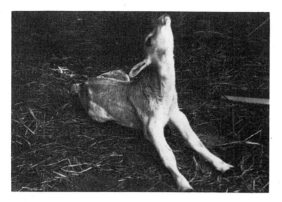

Figure 22 Severe neck retraction in thiamine deficiency (From Zaechi, Acta. Vet. Med. Napoli. *8*, 1962).

DEFICIENCY OF THIAMINE IN HUMANS

A number of experimental thiamine depletion studies have been undertaken over the past 20 years (see also p. 9 and Figure 3). Such depletion leads in man to well marked mental symptoms which include depression, irritability, failure to concentrate and defective memory. Subjective and objective changes in the peripheral nervous system were encountered including tenderness of the calf muscles, partial anaesthesia, muscle weakness (particularly of lower limbs) paraesthesia and hyperaesthesia, reduced or absent tendon reflexes. Electro-cardiographical changes showed the development of a cardiomyopathy. More general complaints included asthenia, loss of weight, anorexia and gastric upsets.

Although the majority of the changes were reversed after administration of thiamine, some irreversible peripheral nervous system changes occurred.

Vitamin B_1 deficiency may arise naturally either directly as a result of low intake of the vitamin or from disproportionate carbohydrate ingestion. During pregnancy increased tissue utilization may cause a deficiency which is often aggravated by loss of appetite and vomiting. Diseases interfering with absorption such as chronic ulcerative colitis and sprue may also produce deficiency even when the dietary intake is adequate. A major cause of thiamine deficiency in industrially developed communities is chronic alcoholism.

Although frank beri-beri is relatively rare in Europe, minor degrees of deficiency causing listlessness, apprehension, anorexia and fatigue are not uncommon. Manual dexterity may be lost and the patient often becomes irritable, confused and inattentive to detail.

Gross deficiency of vitamin B_1 gives rise to the condition known as 'beri-beri' and since the vitamin is intimately connected with general metabolism, all types of tissue may be affected. Signs and symptoms vary, depending upon the individual, the duration and severity of the deficiency and the abruptness of onset. Thus there are three main types of beri-beri –

neuritic, 'dry' (Figure 23), cardiac oedematous, 'wet' (Figure 24) or cerebral beri-beri (Wernicke's syndrome and possibly Korsakoff's psychosis). Cerebral symptoms, often with profound mental changes, are particularly likely to follow sudden severe deficiency. Other manifestations are more common if the deficiency is chronic.

Infantile beri-beri is usually acute in onset. The infant is disinclined to feed, there may be abdominal distension and tenderness accompanied by colicky pain and vomiting, constipation and diminished excretion of urine. Oedema may cause an abnormal increase in weight. Later symptoms include tachycardia, raised respiratory rate, dyspnoea and signs of heart failure often accompanied by clinical evidence of gross cardiac enlargement.

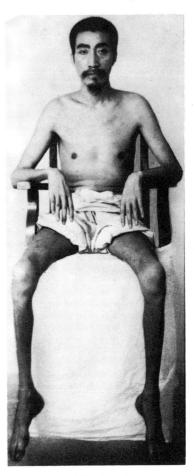

The early symptoms of B$_1$ deficiency are anorexia and vomiting and these, together with impaired absorption, form a vicious circle which, once established, produces a rapid deterioration in the patient's condition. The subject becomes easily fatigued and loses weight and vigour. Nystagmus is a valuable early diagnostic sign in cerebral beri-beri. Peripheral neuritic pain, tachycardia, palpitation and dyspnoea on exertion are noticed early.

Other outstanding symptoms include oedema, intermittent tenderness of the calf muscles, skin hyperaesthesia or anaesthesia, disappearance of the vibration sense and of ankle jerks. In the extreme stage of deficiency, there is muscle wasting, foot-drop and wrist-drop, paralysis, cardiac enlargement and circulatory failure.

Recent studies suggest that some degree of thiamine deficiency is widespread in the elderly.

A useful sign of mild and moderate thiamine deficiency is myotactic irritability (Plate 9).

Figure 23 'Dry' beri-beri showing wrist-drop, foot-drop and marked wasting of lower extremities.

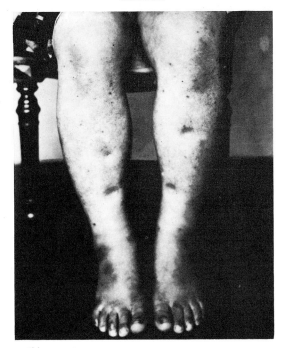

Figure 24 'Wet' beri-beri, showing extensive oedema of the legs.

THERAPY

Deficiency state

Vitamin B_1 is specific in the treatment of beri-beri and other conditions associated with vitamin B_1 deficiency.

Vitamin B_1 deficiency is frequently involved in the aetiology of peripheral neuritis, and treatment with the vitamin may also prove useful in neuritis due to other causes. Neuritis accompanying alcoholism and pregnancy responds particularly well to vitamin B_1 therapy. In delirium tremens, large doses of vitamin B_1 combined with other vitamins should be given by injection.

In cardiac disease B_1 therapy is generally only of value when the condition is associated with a known deficiency, but minor deficiencies are probably more common than is generally suspected. In mild deficiency states a daily dose of 10 mg is usually sufficient but this is increased up to 50 mg in severe cases.

Other disorders

Although at present there is no rational explanation for their use, large doses of the vitamin (50–600 mg daily) have been recommended in the treatment of such painful conditions as lumbago, sciatica, trigeminal neuralgia, facial paralysis and optic neuritis. The author has seen such cases treated with success.

TOXICITY

Signs of overdosage have not been noted; however, it is recognized that an anaphylactic reaction may sometimes occur after an *injection* of B_1, probably due to sensitization to the vitamin. Because of this injections of B_1 should not be given intravenously, except in the case of comatose patients who may be given large doses of vitamins by slow intravenous drip.

Riboflavine

Vitamin B₂ Lactoflavine

The fact that a growth-promoting factor remained after heat destruction of the anti-neuritic factor in yeast extracts was first noted in 1920 by Emmett. This was designated vitamin B_2. In 1932 Warburg and Christian described a new oxidative enzyme in yeast and one year later the two were established as identical. The constitution and the chemical synthesis were both elucidated in 1935.

CHEMISTRY

The structural formula of riboflavine is shown at the beginning of the chapter. Chemically it is an isoalloxazine derivative with a ribitol side chain. The synonym lactoflavine refers to its presence in milk.

It consists of orange-yellow crystals which melt at about 280°C with decomposition. It is thermostable at ordinary temperatures and unaffected by atmospheric oxygen. It is very slightly soluble in water, the solution exhibiting a strong yellow-green fluorescence. It is insoluble in organic solvents, stable in strongly acid solution, unstable in the presence of alkali, or when exposed to light or ultraviolet radiation.

SOURCES

The content of riboflavine in various foodstuffs is shown in Table 16. Riboflavine is widely distributed in all leafy vegetables, in the flesh of warm blooded animals and in fish.

Table 16 Content of riboflavine in certain foods.

	Riboflavine mg/100g
Wholemeal flour	0·1–0·2
White flour	0·04–0·08
Brown bread	0·09
White bread	0·07
Rice, polished	0·03
treated by parboiling	0·06–0·09
Spinach	0·2–0·4
Beans	0·18
Blackcurrants	0·05
Cows milk	0·14–0·18
Cheese	0·3–0·7
Lean meat (pork, beef)	0·1–0·3
Eggs (each)	0·4

REQUIREMENTS

Riboflavine can be synthesized by bacteria within the intestinal tract of many species but human entero-synthesis is not sufficient to meet the whole requirements. The daily requirement for riboflavine may be related to the intensity of metabolism but the evidence is not conclusive. For human beings the daily requirements are shown in Table 17 based generally on 0·6

Table 17 Daily requirements for riboflavine in humans expressed in mg/day.

		Riboflavine mg/day
Adults		
Man	Sedentary	1·2
	Moderately active	1·4
	Very active	1·6
Woman	Sedentary	1·1
	Moderately active	1·3
	Very active	1·4
	Pregnancy	1·6
	Lactation	2·0
Children		
Both sexes	Under 1 year	0·6
	1–3 years	0·9
	4–6 years	1·2
	7–9 years	1·5
	10–12 years	1·5
Boys	13–15 years	1·8
	16–20 years	1·8
Girls	13–15 years	1·6
	16–20 years	1·6

mg/1000 kcal. The optimum for various animal species is shown in Table 36 (page 194).

METABOLISM

Riboflavine is phosphorylated in the intestinal mucosa during absorption. It is stored in small quantities, in the liver, spleen, kidney and cardiac muscle. These depots are maintained, and even in severe deficiency states, depot riboflavine levels remain at a normal value.

Riboflavine is eliminated in the urine. Daily losses amount to up to 30 per cent of the intake. Small losses occur in the sweat.

Anti-riboflavine action has been found in analogues containing other sugar alcohols in place of the ribityl group, e.g. galactityl. Changing the pyrimidine ring to a 2:4 dinitrobenzene ring also gave a powerful anti-riboflavine activity.

PHYSIOLOGY

Riboflavine can combine in the form of the phosphoric acid ester in the tissues to form two co-enzymes, flavine mononucleotide (FMN) and a flavine-adenine dinucleotide FAD. These in turn can form the prosthetic groups of several different enzyme systems. These enzyme groups with the prosthetic groups (so called flavoproteins) are all concerned with hydrogen transport.

The dinucleotide (FAD) forms the prosthetic group of the following hydrogen transport enzyme systems.

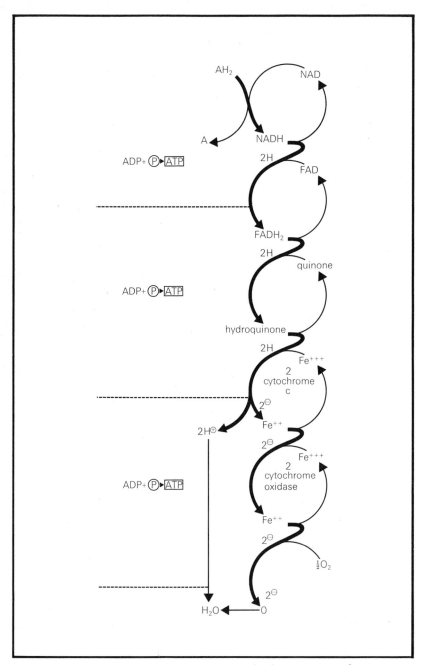

Figure 25 Part played by flavoproteins and quinone in the electron transport chain.

1 Flavoprotein accessory redox systems.

(a) Acting as a link between the pyridine nucleotide systems and the cytochromes. Two of these are specific systems for the reoxidation of the reduced forms of nicotinamide adenine dinucleotide (NAD) and nicotinamide adenine dinucleotide phosphate (NADP).

(b) Acting as a link between the intermediary metabolite and the cytochrome systems; e.g. succinic dehydrogenase important in the tricarboxylic acid cycle, butyryl-co-enzyme A dehydrogenase containing copper as an essential component and the whole range of acyl co-enzyme A dehydrogenases which contain iron and dehydrogenate C_4–C_{16} acyl derivatives as the first step in the β-oxidation of fatty acids.

Flavoprotein containing enzymes thus have an integral role in the biological oxidation reactions of the electron transport chain at various stages. Both FAD and FMN are involved. During these reactions the hydrogen released by the dehydrogenases is converted to water with energy production which is stored as ATP.

A single concept of the present view of this electron transport chain is shown in Figure 25.

2 Oxidase flavoproteins. These carry hydrogen directly to molecular oxygen.

(a) Xanthine oxidase oxidizing hypoxanthine through xanthine to uric acid. This is a dual function enzyme and also oxidizes many aldehydes, including vitamin A aldehyde, to the corresponding carboxylic acids.

(b) Amino acid oxidases.

These oxidize α amino acids to the corresponding imino acids which decompose giving ammonia and a keto acid. There are distinct enzymes oxidizing D amino acids (prosthetic group FAD) and L amino acids (prosthetic group FMN). The specific enzyme glycine dehydrogenase has FAD as its prosthetic group.

Whereas vitamin B_2 is present in most animal organs as a phosphate or a flavine-adenine dinucleotide, the retina of the eyes contains free vitamin B_2 in relatively large amounts. The function it fulfils there, however, is still not clear. In avascular tissues such as the cornea it is thought that oxidation takes place by means of a riboflavine-containing enzyme. In deficiency of the vitamin the body attempts oxygenation by vascularization.

In both animals and man riboflavine is essential to growth and life. It is in fact surprising, in view of its widespread metabolic function, that more florid symptoms are not seen during riboflavine deprivation.

DEFICIENCY OF RIBOFLAVINE IN ANIMALS

The typical symptoms of an early deficiency first appear in the skin and mucous membranes, and especially in the form of inflammation at the transition points between the two in the region of the body apertures. Such early symptoms are inflammation of the mouth and nasal mucous membranes, the corners of the mouth and eye-lids. The inflammation of the mucous membranes also frequently includes the genital tract. Atrophy, oedema and inflammation of the mucous membranes of the digestive tract result in difficulties in swallowing, disorders in food absorption and diarrhoea in pigs, dogs and fowl. In the case of turkeys, typical signs are inflammation of the skin at the extremities and crustiness forming around the beak.

Inflammation of the conjunctiva is a particularly characteristic symptom of a deficiency of riboflavine in horses. Deposits of pigment are to be found in the iris and result in disturbed vision; moreover, clouding of the cornea and sensitivity to light are typical indications of riboflavine deficiency. In veterinary practice the syndrome is known as periodic ophthalmia.

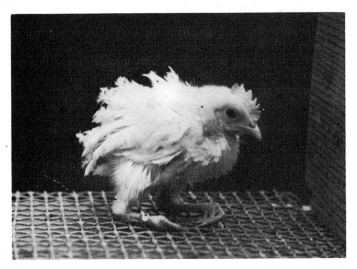

Figure 26 Typical curled toe paralysis in a fowl with riboflavine deficiency (By courtesy of Dr. C. R. Gran, Div. of Agric. Science, University of California).

In the liver there is a fatty infiltration, this is most marked in dogs ('yellow liver'). The kidneys show congestion and haemorrhages. General muscular debility, trembling, awkward movements and signs of paralysis, occur in riboflavine deficiency. Curled toe paralysis in chicks is particularly characteristic (Figure 26). In new-born animals where the mothers suffered from B_2 deficiency, skeletal abnormalities are frequent, e.g. shortened bones, fused ribs, syndactylism, cleft palate. Typical damage to the nerve tissue in both birds and mammals consists of a myelin degeneration in the region of the peripheral nerve roots, pyramidal tracts and cranial nerves which manifests itself in the form of ataxia and cramp. As a result of riboflavine deficiency, foetal resorption, sterility, premature births and stillbirths are observed. In laying poultry, hatchability of incubated eggs is first reduced and subsequently egg production falls. The bone marrow shows an erythroid hypoplasia and in consequence of this an aplastic type of anaemia.

DEFICIENCY OF RIBOFLAVINE IN HUMANS

Early symptoms of riboflavine deficiency may be general in nature, or may be related to oral or ocular lesions. Soreness and burning of the lips, mouth and tongue are common complaints and this is usually accompanied by discomfort in eating and swallowing. Ocular symptoms include photophobia, lachrymation, burning and itching of the eyes, visual fatigue, blepharospasm and loss of visual acuity which cannot be accounted for by refractive error. A sensation of 'grittiness' under the lids is often present.

Lesions of the lips begin with pallor and maceration at the angles of the mouth or with dryness, redness and denudation along the line of closure. In severe deficiency ulceration may occur, and at the angles transverse fissures appear which may extend outwards for a centimetre or more. The

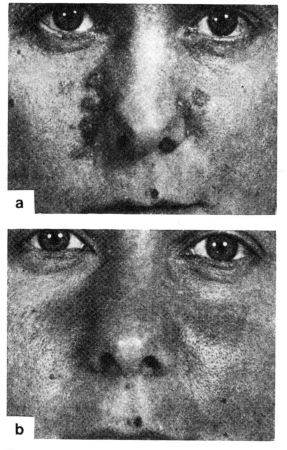

Figure 27
(a) Recurrent bilateral eczema of the nose and naso-labial folds.
(b) Response to riboflavine.

lesions of the lips have been designated 'cheilosis' and those at the angles of the mouth 'angular stomatitis' (Plate 13). There is still some dispute about the tongue signs particularly in relation to distinguishing between the glossitis of riboflavine and nicotinic acid deficiency. In practice the two are often associated (see also page 162).

The early case, many experts believe on therapeutic grounds, manifests itself as the 'geographical tongue' (Plate 12b). There is a circular loss of filiform papillae, with enlargement of fungiform papillae giving a pebbled appearance. In a more advanced case there is complete shedding of the filiform papillae, accentuated fungiform papillae at the tip of the tongue and extensive fissuring (Plate 14).

The dermatitis due to riboflavine deficiency begins most often in the nasolabial fold and is scaly and oily in character (Figure 27). Similar lesions may also appear around the eyes and on the ears. Dermatitis of the scrotum or vulva is frequently present.

The eye lesions of ariboflavinosis have been the subject of extensive investigation but are still a matter of controversy.

A characteristic vascularization of the cornea has been described, in which capillaries of the limbic plexus proliferate and extend into the superficial layers of the cornea anastomosing to form tiers or loops (Plate 15). Corneal vascularization due to riboflavine deficiency always occurs in the entire circumference of the cornea and is nearly always bilateral. Circumcorneal injection may represent the initial stages of corneal vascularization but is, in itself, quite non-specific. Corneal opacities may develop. The bone marrow shows an erythroid hypoplasia and as a consequence of this an aplastic type of anaemia develops.

A theory has now been advanced which might explain the varying and apparently non-specific nature of the abnormalities accompanying ariboflavinosis. It is based upon the fact that riboflavine is necessary for growth.

As any local trauma must be replaced by new growth it is suggested that the location of signs of deficiency would depend upon the presence of local irritation, infection etc. In some cases the precipitating factor may be obvious as in angular stomatitis after herpes simplex; in other instances it may not. The results of animal experiments have lent substance to this point of view.

In practice a combination of several of the signs and symptoms enumerated above and the knowledge that the patient has been subsisting on an inadequate diet, or has a defect in absorption, should lead to correct diagnosis of ariboflavinosis. This can be confirmed by response to treatment with the specific vitamin.

THERAPY

Deficiency states

Riboflavine is employed mainly for the treatment of the signs and symptoms of deficiency described above. Oral and skin lesions suggestive of riboflavine deficiency are not uncommon in patients who have undergone total or subtotal gastrectomy, and have been reported in patients being treated with chloramphenicol and other antibiotics. In both instances prophylactic treatment with a vitamin B-complex preparation is probably wise at a dose of 3 mg daily. Established cases should be treated with riboflavine (10–60 mg daily) supplemented by other members of the B-complex; by injection if necessary. Recovery however may be slow.

Other disorders

Surgery or trauma to the eye may precipitate corneal vascularization and, therefore, it is recommended that riboflavine be given prior to ocular surgery, especially if the patient shows any signs of malnutrition. Claims have been made that riboflavine is of value in the treatment of trachomatous pannus, angular blepharitis and phlyctenular keratitis.

Riboflavine is sometimes effective in the treatment of migraine and also of muscle cramps although there is no rationale for any of these uses. 30 mg daily is the usual dose in these disorders.

Pyridoxine

Vitamin B$_6$

The occurrence of a typical pyridoxine deficiency state was first noted in rat experiments on pellagra producing diets in 1926. It was distinguished from the other members of the B complex and designated B_6 in 1934. Isolation, determination of constitution and synthesis were undertaken in 1938–9.

CHEMISTRY

Although the term 'vitamin B_6' is classically applied to pyridoxine, it is probably better to use the term 'B_6' to denote several chemical compounds having vitamin B_6 activity. Under the new terminology pyridoxine is used as a name to cover the 'B_6 group'. These are pyridoxine (new terminology pyridoxol) (the alcohol), its aldehyde (pyridoxal), and its amine (pyridoxamine). They all have the general formula shown at the beginning of the chapter. For pyridoxine (pyridoxol) $R=CH_2OH$; pyridoxal $R=CHO$; pyridoxamine $R=CH_2NH_2$.

These substances are colourless crystals soluble in water and alcohol both as the free bases and the commonly available hydrochlorides. They are resistant to normal heat but are decomposed by alkalis and ultraviolet light. Pyridoxine hydrochloride decomposes at its melting point (204°–206°C).

SOURCES

The three forms are widely distributed in low concentrations in all animal and plant tissues. The chief sources in the diet are shown in Table 18.

Table 18 Content of vitamin B_6 in various foods.

	Vitamin B_6 mg/100 g
Cows milk	0·03–0·3
Cheese	0·04–0·8
Eggs (each)	0·25
Meat (beef, lamb, chicken, pork)	0·08–0·3
Fish (salmon, herring)	0·45
Flour-wholemeal extraction	0·4–0·7
80% ”	0·1–0·3
70% ”	0·08–0·16
Potatoes	0·14–0·23
Spinach	0·22
Peas	0·16
Beans	0·1
Carrots	0·7
Oranges	0·05

REQUIREMENTS

There is no doubt that vitamin B_6 is produced by micro-organisms of the intestinal tracts of animals and man. It appears likely that little if any of this is absorbed and utilized. An adequate human diet for most circumstances is one containing between 1 and 2 mg vitamin B_6 compounds daily (Table

Pyridoxine

Table 19 Daily requirements for pyridoxine in humans expressed in mg/day.

	Pyridoxine mg/day
Adults, male and female	2·0
Pregnancy and lactation	2·5*
Infants	0·4
Children	0·6—2·0

* Figures as high as 10 mg have been suggested.

19). It should however be noted that these values are tentative at present. Estimated requirements for animals are shown in Table 36 (p. 194).

METABOLISM

Very little is known about the factors influencing absorption of B_6 although it is rapidly absorbed. The compound is distributed throughout the animal tissues but in the form of the co-enzyme, and storage of vitamin B_6 as such is not known.

Some 70 per cent of the vitamin is excreted in the urine as the inactive metabolite 4-pyridoxic acid.

Attention has been drawn recently to an anaemia in pyridoxine deficiency in man. This was originally encountered in a group of patients receiving a pyridoxine deficient diet and an antagonist. Certain cases with anaemia in association with kwashiorkor or marasmus however appear to respond, at least partially, to pyridoxine.

The anaemia is microcytic hypochromic in type and the marrow showed hypoplasia akin to that seen in animals with riboflavine deficiency (see also page 99).

PHYSIOLOGY

The B_6 group are rapidly converted in the body into the co-enzymes pyridoxal phosphate and pyridoxamine phosphate. These co-enzymes play an essential role in protein metabolism. Pyridoxal phosphate forms the prosthetic group of the following enzymes:

1 Transaminases. The mode of action is probably as an amino group transfer mechanism by the formation of pyridoxamine. The reaction allows the transfer of amino groups from glutamic and aspartic acid to certain α-keto acids. Thus synthesis of amino acids is possible from carbohydrate intermediates e.g.

(a) Glutamic acid+pyruvic acid=α-ketoglutaric acid+ alanine.

(b) Glutamic acid+oxaloacetic acid=α-ketoglutaric acid+aspartic acid.

In other transaminase reactions either glutamine or aspargine, can act directly as the amino donor to pyridoxal phosphate-containing enzymes. Transamination plays an essential role in urea formation by providing aspartic acid, one of the amino donors.

2 Codecarboxylases $RCHNH_2COOH \rightarrow RCH_2NH_2 + CO_2$. Several en-

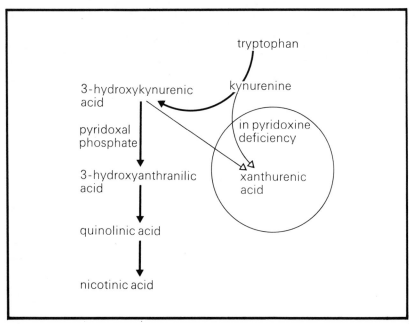

Figure 28 Pyridoxal phosphate dependent stage of synthesis of nicotinic acid from trypto-phan.

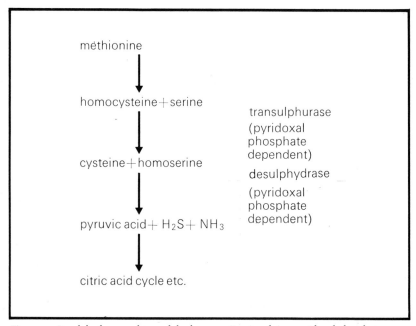

Figure 29 Desulphydrases and transulphydrase reaction involving pyridoxal phosphate.

zymes specific for the decarboxylation of amino acids have been found in animal tissues. These all appear to be pyridoxal phosphate dependent. Substrates include glutamic acid, tyrosine, histidine, cysteic acid and amino acid derivatives, e.g. 5-hydroxytryptophan. The decarboxylases convert them into the physiologically important amines (Table 20).

Table 20 Biologically important amines derived from amino acids or amino acid derivatives under the action of decarboxylase.

Amino acid	Amine
Histidine	Histamine
5-Hydroxy tryptophan	5-Hydroxytryptamine (Serotonin)
Aspartic acid	β-Alanine
Glutamic acid	γ-Aminobutyric acid
Phenylalanine	⎧ Noradrenaline
Tyrosine	⎨ Adrenaline
	⎪ Tyramine
	⎩ Dopamine
Cysteic acid	Taurine

3 Kynureninase. In pyridoxine deficiency the production of nicotinic acid from tryptophan is impaired at the hydroxykynurenine stage (Figure 28). This compound instead of being converted to hydroxyanthranilic acid forms xanthurenic acid, the urinary excretion of which has been used as a biochemical index of inadequate pyridoxine.

4 Deaminases. For serine, threonine and cystathionine (acts also on homoserine).

5 Desulphydrases and transulphurases in the interconversion and metabolism of sulphur containing amino acids (Figure 29).

(a) Desulphydrase on cysteine.

(b) Transulphurases. In the synthesis of cystine-through cysteine. The sulphydryl group of homocysteine (derived by demethylation of methionine) is transferred to the carbon chain of serine.

6 In the conversion of linoleic to arachidonic acid in the metabolism of essential fatty acids.

7 Biosynthesis of co-enzyme A, which is impaired in vitamin B_6 deficiency.

8 Glycogen phosphorylase which catalyses the breakdown of glycogen reserves to give glucose-1-phosphate in muscle and liver.

9 Threonine aldolase.

10 The formation of δ-amino laevulinic acid from succinyl Co A and glycine. This is the first step in porphyrin synthesis.

11 Transmethylation by methionine.

12 Incorporation of iron in haemoglobin synthesis.

As a result of these reactions pyridoxal phosphate forms an essential enzyme for energy production (supplying metabolites to the Kreb's cycle), fat metabolism, central nervous system activity, and haemoglobin production.

Pyridoxine the co-enzyme for decarboxylation of amino acid has an important part to play in the brain metabolism. In particular it is required for the formation of the whole group of brain amines which probably act as synaptic transmitters in various brain areas (noradrenaline, adrenaline, tyramine, dopamine, and serotonin-5 hydroxytryptamine). But not only is it a cofactor in the production of these amines of 'brain facilitation' but also of the widely scattered inhibitory brain amine γ-amino butyric acid. Experience suggests that pyridoxine is a cofactor in a rate limiting stage of the production of γ-amino butyric acid but not of the other brain amines.

Two main antagonists have been described for several animal species: desoxypyridoxine and the tuberculostatic drug isoniazid.

In addition to these two substances, antagonism has also been reported with hydrallazine (antihypertensive) and penicillamine (used in the treatment of the rare Wilson's disease).

Interference with vitamin B_6 functions by these drugs is often sufficiently severe to produce both biochemical and clinical defects—predominantly neuritis and convulsions.

When pyridoxine hydrochloride is administered to patients who are receiving levodopa for relief of parkinsonism it nullifies the effect of levodopa on the central nervous system.

DEFICIENCY OF VITAMIN B_6 IN ANIMALS

Vitamin B_6 has proved to be an essential growth factor for all experimental and domestic animals so far investigated. The exact manifestations vary from one species to another but the main effects are:

1 Some loss of appetite, poor food utilization and weight loss or poor weight gain; vomiting; diarrhoea.

2 'Acrodynia' characterized by hyperkeratosis and acanthosis of the ears, paws (Figure 30), snout and tail, and oedema of the corium. This condition appears to be identical with that due to lack of certain unsaturated fatty

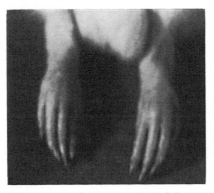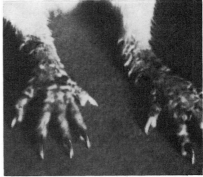

Figure 30 Acrodynia in vitamin B_6 deficient rat (right) compared with normal.

acids and although the exact inter-relationship is not known it is believed that fat exerts a sparing action on pyridoxine.

3 Paralysis of the hind extremities at first, followed by a progressive degeneration of the peripheral nerves with ataxia and paralysis. Finally, convulsions occur at irregular intervals prior to death.

4 A brown secretion around the eyes and a flow of tears with a weakening of vision until complete blindness is reached.

5 The blood picture shows a microcytic hypochromic anaemia.

Vitamin B$_6$ deficiency manifests itself in fowl in much the same way as it does in mammals (Figure 31). In chickens, turkeys and ducks, the following symptoms are described: loss of appetite, poor growth, dermatitis, marked anaemia and convulsions. Egg output and fertility are considerably impaired in vitamin B$_6$ deficiency.

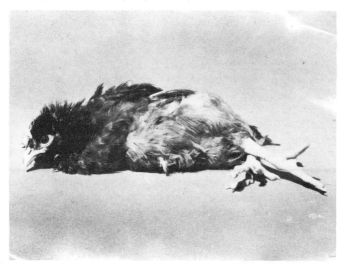

Figure 31 Chick showing advanced vitamin B$_6$ deficiency. Nervous disorders, stiff extremities, inability to stand.

In ruminants, clinical symptoms are naturally rare due to the synthesis in the fore stomach which covers their requirement, but in calves and lambs where the ruminant stomach is not fully developed, the same symptoms occur with a deficient diet as in other animals.

In monkeys, deficiency causes arteriosclerotic lesions which bear a close resemblance to those of human arteriosclerosis. Caries is also found in pyridoxine deficient monkeys. The evidence linking this observation with human caries is inconclusive.

DEFICIENCY OF VITAMIN B$_6$ IN HUMANS

Although recent work suggests that little of the pyridoxine synthesized by intestinal bacteria is absorbed, it has proved difficult to induce deficiency symptoms by dietary restriction. The administration of the pyridoxine antagonist desoxypyridoxine has been used to produce symptoms due to interference with pyridoxine function in human volunteers who were on a pyridoxine depleted diet. Seborrhoea-like lesions developed about the eyes, nose and mouth and some subjects showed cheilosis and glossitis. A depression of the lymphocyte count was a fairly constant finding. Doubt has been cast, however, on whether an antagonist produced syndrome mimics the natural deficiency disease. The major findings, when a pyridoxine deficient diet alone was employed, were a hypochromic anaemia and loss of ability to convert tryptophan to nicotinic acid.

The peripheral neuritis occurring in patients under treatment with large doses of isoniazid is probably due to impairment of the efficiency of vitamin B_6 enzymes.

Concern has recently been expressed over the pyridoxine status during pregnancy and while taking steroid contraceptive pills. There is biochemical evidence of deficiency under each of these circumstances but no clear evidence of physical manifestations (apart possibly from malaise). On general principles, however, higher intake is advisable.

Recently, several cases of pyridoxine deficiency in infants have been described due to inadequate commercial milk formulae. The characteristic feature in these infants has been convulsions, probably due to brain γ-amino butyric acid depletion.

An interesting recent discovery has been a group of disorders which have been termed collectively 'vitamin B_6 dependency states'. In these patients tissue levels of pyridoxine are normal but there is impairment of the cofactor binding site on the apoenzyme, which therefore cannot function adequately. The clinical picture depends on the enzyme involved (Table 21) but all are inherited defects ('inborn error of metabolism'). They can be relieved by the administration of adequate amounts of pyridoxine.

Table 21 Pyridoxine dependent-syndromes and their biochemical features.

Disease	Clinical findings	Probable abnormal enzyme	Biochemical findings
Infantile seizures (some)	Fits	Glutamic acid decarboxylase	Decreased brain G.A.B.A.
Pyridoxine responsive anaemia (some)	Hypochromic anaemia	δ-aminolavulinic acid synthetase	Defective heme synthesis
Familial xanthurenic acid	Urticaria	Kynureninase	Xanthurenic acid-uria
Cystathioninuria	Mental retardation	Cystathioninase	Cystathioninuria

THERAPY

Deficiency states

A true deficiency state due to inadequate diet is rarely seen. Pyridoxine in doses of 40–150 mg per day is given in peripheral neuritis due to treat ment with isoniazid and related compounds and in pyridoxine dependency states. Some cases of cheilosis respond best to pyridoxine, as do some cases of hypochromic anaemia. The neurological symptoms associated with pellagra and beri-beri are said to be improved with pyridoxine.

Pyridoxine appears to be required in increased amounts during pregnancy and while taking steroid contraceptive pills, and it is used in the treatment of hyperemesis gravidarum (dose 100–200 mg/day).

Other disorders

Pyridoxine has been used (up to 300 mg/day) for the prevention and treatment of nausea and vomiting due to irradiation, drug therapy, anaesthesia and in travel sickness but a good response is not always seen. It has also been recommended for the treatment of agranulocytosis but this latter use will not stand critical examination. It has been suggested that topically applied pyridoxine cures patients with the sicca type of seborrhoeic dermatitis.

Nicotinic Acid
Niacin, Pellagra-Preventive (P.P.) factor

Pellagra has been recognized as a disease since the eighteenth century in Italy. In 1912 Funk postulated a pellagra preventive vitamin. In 1926 pellagra was induced in volunteers by a deficient diet and both these volunteers and patients were cured with yeast. The isolation of nicotinic acid was accomplished in 1912 from yeast and its identity with the P.P. factor established in 1937.

CHEMISTRY

Nicotinic acid is pyridine β-carboxylic acid (R=OH in the illustration); nicotinamide is the corresponding amide (R=NH$_2$). Both nicotinic acid and nicotinamide are white crystalline solids soluble in water. They are not heat labile, nor are they sensitive to light, air or alkalis. Since both are equiactive as vitamins terminology in the literature is often confused and P.P. factor or niacin are often used as group names.

Unless specifically mentioned in the section nicotinic acid has been used as the representative member of the pair.

SOURCES

Nicotinic acid is present in the most varied foodstuffs apart from actual fatty substances, and is in particularly rich supply in meat, fish, wheat and wheat wholemeal. It is often present in the food in a form which is not absorbable. This is particularly true of maize and severe deficiency of nicotinic acid occurs primarily in areas of the world where maize is the main article of diet. It occurs in Mexico less frequently than one might expect; there it is the custom – obviously resulting from centuries of experience – to treat the maize with limewater before making 'tortillas' and in this way, the nicotinic acid is liberated.

The levels of nicotinic acid in dietary ingredients are shown in Table 22.

Table 22 Content of nicotinic acid in various foods.

	Nicotinic acid mg/100 g
Meat (beef, pork)	4·0–5·8
Fish	2·0–11
Eggs (each)	0·03 mg
Cows milk	0·07–0·4
Cheese	1–2
Wheat flour, wholemeal	4·8–5·5
80% extraction	0·9–1·1
70% extraction	0·7–0·8
Maize flour	2·0
Potatoes	0·9
Broccoli	0·9
Tomatoes	0·9
Carrots	0·7

REQUIREMENTS

At one time it was believed that biosynthesis of nicotinic acid from trypto-phan occurred in the intestine by bacterial action. It now appears that intestinal production is only of minor importance in the human. On the other hand true biosynthesis of nicotinic acid from tryptophan occurs, but probably only a small fraction of dietary tryptophan is used thus.

The value of tryptophan as a preliminary stage for nicotinic acid depends not only on the tryptophan intake but also upon other essential amino acids such as leucine, isoleucine, valine, threonine and lysine and vitamins such as vitamin B_1, vitamin B_6 and biotin contained in the diet.

There is inadequate experimental evidence on which to base accurate recommended levels of intake but in general it appears that the intake for adults should be about 6·5 mg/1000 kcal but with a minimum of 13 mg. Increased intake is advisable in pregnancy and lactation. Details are shown in Table 23.

Table 23 Daily requirements for nicotinic acid in humans expressed in mg/day.

		Nicotinic acid mg/day*
Adults		
Man	Sedentary	16
	Moderately active	17
	Very active	18
Woman	Sedentary	12
	Moderately active	13
	Very active	14
	Pregnancy 1st half	14
	2nd half	15
	Lactation	17
Children		
Both sexes	Under 1 year	6
	1–3 years	9
	4–6 years	11
	7–9 years	14
	10–12 years	16
Boys	13–15 years	18
	16–20 years	20
Girls	13–15 years	14
	16–20 years	16

*Expressed as equivalents of the preformed vitamin and the precursor, tryptophan: 60 mg tryptophan represents 1 mg nicotinic acid.

These requirements can be met in part from the tryptophan intake: 60 mg tryptophan being equivalent to 1 mg nicotinic acid. The main stages in the biosynthesis are shown in Figure 28 (page 96).

Estimated requirements for animals are shown in Table 36 (page 194).

METABOLISM

Intestinal absorption of nicotinic acid is normally very efficient. The compound is converted in the body into the co-enzymes and, though these are widely distributed, no true storage occurs.

A small amount of nicotinic acid or nicotinamide is excreted. The largest proportion is excreted as N-methyl nicotinamide.

In animals the principal antagonist that has been studied is 3-acetyl-pyridine.

Although not a direct antagonist, the presence of leucine increases the requirement of nicotinic acid. This amino acid is found in high concentration in millet. In India, where millet forms a high proportion of the diet, nicotinic acid deficiency is likely to occur due to the leucine.

PHYSIOLOGY

Nicotinic acid as the amide is an indispensable component of the hydrogen-carrying co-enzymes. These are: co-enzyme I-nicotinamide adenine dinucleotide (NAD) (old terminology – diphosphopyridine nucleotide, DPN) and co-enzyme II-nicotinamide adenine dinucleotide phosphate (NADP) (previously called triphosphopyridine nucleotide, TPN). In both these co-enzymes, nicotinamide represents the effective group which participates directly in the transfer of hydrogen.

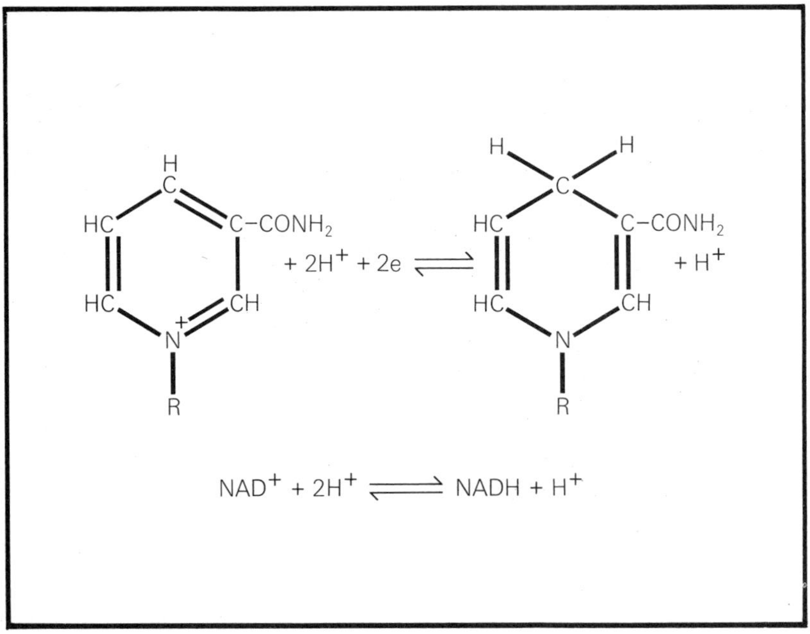

Figure 32 Hydrogen acceptor function of nicotinamide containing co-enzymes. R=adenine dinucleotide (=NAD):=adenine dinucleotide phosphate (=NADP).

106

The transfer of hydrogen catalysed by co-enzymes I and II plays a decisive role in intermediary metabolism.

It is believed that the hydrogen acceptor function of these two co-enzymes resides in the para position of the nicotinamide component (Figure 32). This reaction occurs as a co-enzyme function with the majority of de-hydrogenases. The classical situation for this is in the energy production pathway (see Figure 25, page 86).

Table 24 Dehydrogenases requiring:

NAD	NADP
Soluble	
α-glycerophosphate	
Lactic (and hence in	Glucose-6-phosphate
pyruvate metabolism)	
Malic	D-iso-Citric (in mitochondria)
D-glyceraldehyde	Malic decarboxylase
phosphate	
β-hydroxybutyric	SH-glutathione
Glucose	NAD-H
L-Glutamic	FAD-H
β-Hydroxy	
fatty-acyl-CoA	
NADP-H	
FAD-H	

A list of some of the most important dehydrogenases using NAD or NADP co-enzymes is shown in Table 24. In addition to these, NAD is used as co-enzyme by UDP-D-glucose 4^1-epimerase, a system by which galactose 1−P is converted to glucose 1−P and hence to glycogen.

The biochemical functions are of paramount importance for normal tissue integrity, and particularly for the skin, the gastrointestinal tract and the nervous system.

In addition to these reactions, nicotinic acid, but not the amide, has two pharmacological actions:

1 Peripheral vasodilation.
2 Serum cholesterol reducing properties.

DEFICIENCY OF NICOTINIC ACID IN ANIMALS
A deficiency of nicotinic acid is characterized by severe metabolic disorders in the skin and the digestive organs.

The first signs to appear are loss of appetite, retarded growth (Figure 33), weakness, digestive disorders and diarrhoea. The mucous membranes of the digestive tract are inflamed; necrosis, ulcers and bleeding develop in the large intestine and the caecum. The coat is rough and a scaly dermatitis forms. A microcytic anaemia develops.

In dogs there is a typical red, and later dark blue, pigmentation of the

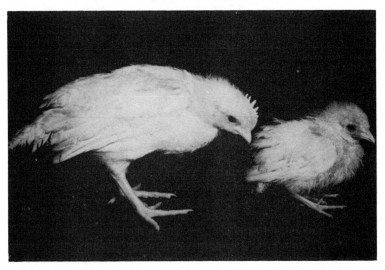

Figure 33 Retarded growth and poor feathering of a chick with nicotinic acid deficiency compared with a normal chick of the same age (By courtesy of Dr. C. A. Elvehjem, University of Wisconsin, Dept. of Biochemistry).

tongue ('black tongue') and viscous, ill-smelling saliva is secreted. In some species (dogs and cats) degenerative changes are found in the epithelium of the testes. They also suffer from degeneration in the nervous system which manifests itself as ataxia, disturbed reflexes, paralysis and epileptic attacks.

Characteristic features in poultry are an enlargement of the spring joint and a curved femur.

DEFICIENCY OF NICOTINIC ACID IN HUMANS

Nicotinic acid deficiency is one of the major factors in the development of pellagra, hence the synonym P.P. (pellgra-preventive) factor. The symptoms of pellagra vary considerably and are often summarized in the mnemonic 'Diarrhoea, Dermatitis and Dementia'. The gastrointestinal symptoms are often the first to appear and include glossitis and stomatitis, the tongue having a characteristic swollen and 'beefy-red' appearance (Plate 7). There is also anorexia, abdominal discomfort and

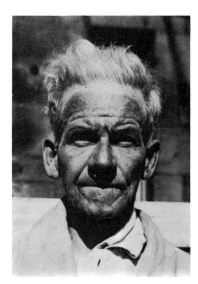

Figure 34 Pellagrous pigmentation of the face in a patient in this country. Note the pale area which was covered by the hat.

108

diarrhoea. Pellagrous dermatitis has a characteristic 'symmetrical' appearance and is usually confined to parts of the body exposed to light or trauma (Figure 35). The lesions are precipitated by exposure to sunlight (Figure 34), fires and radiant heat. Although severe desquamating lesions are occasionally seen, diagnosis is now made more commonly at an earlier stage. Early mental symptoms include lassitude, apprehension, depression and loss of memory and these may be succeeded by disorientation, confusion, hysteria and sometimes maniacal outbursts. Pellagra sine pellagra is the description sometimes applied to the disease in the absence of cutaneous manifestations.

A condition characterized by an encephalopathic syndrome closely related to Wernicke's encephalopathy is believed to result from acute nicotinic acid deficiency. The clinical picture includes clouding of consciousness, cog-wheel rigidity and uncontrollable sucking and grasping reflexes. Other symptoms such as oculomotor disturbances, stupor, delirium, and agitated depression have been described.

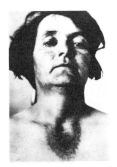
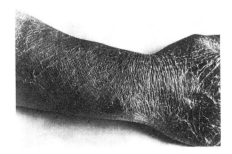
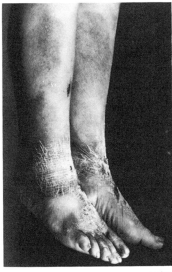

Figure 35 Pellagra dermatitis seen in this country in an elderly woman. Note characteristic changes in hands and feet and Casal's necklace.

Pellagra is probably not a simple nicotinic acid deficiency syndrome and deficiency of several additional factors including members of the vitamin B-complex may also be involved. It is endemic in maize-eating areas and may occur even when the diet appears to be adequate with respect to nicotinic acid.

THERAPY

Deficiency states

Nicotinamide (or nicotinic acid) is specific in the treatment of the glossitis, dermatitis and alimentary and mental symptoms seen in pellagra. The peripheral neuritis and the ocular symptoms commonly associated with this condition respond more readily to vitamin B_1 and riboflavine respectively. In addition, nicotinamide has been used in the treatment of a number of other diseases which involve the gastrointestinal tract, such as the sprue syndrome, and in glossitis and stomatitis due to various causes. For prophylaxis doses up to 50 mg daily are given. For therapy the daily dose in a severe pellagra may be up to 500 mg.

OTHER DISORDERS

The vasodilator properties of nicotinic acid have been employed in the treatment of various conditions where vasospasm may be considered to be part of the syndrome (dose 100–300 mg/day).

High doses of nicotinic acid (1–3 g per day) have been used successfully for cholesterol reduction.

Similar high doses have been advocated in the therapy of acute schizophrenia, but careful studies do not substantiate the early enthusiastic reports.

Folic Acid

Vitamin M; Lactobacillus casei factor:
Vitamin B$_c$; P.G.A.; Folacin

An anti-anaemic factor for monkeys was found in yeast and liver concentrates and designated vitamin M in 1935. In 1939 an anti-anaemic factor for chicks was found in liver and called vitamin B_c. One year later a growth factor for *Lactobacillus casei* was found: in the same year a growth factor for *Streptococcus lactis* was found in spinach and named folic acid. In the mid-1940s these were all found to be the same substance, and determination of its constitution and synthesis was accomplished.

CHEMISTRY

Folacin is now used as the group name to distinguish naturally occurring compounds of this class, the pure substance being designated pteroylmonoglutamic acid. Since the old name folic acid is still so widely used it is preferred for this chapter.

Folic acid is a yellowish-orange crystalline powder, tasteless and odourless, insoluble in alcohol and ether and other organic solvents. It is slightly soluble in hot water. It has a characteristic ultraviolet absorption spectrum.

Pure folic acid (pteroylglutamic acid) has the structural formula shown at the beginning of the chapter. It is a combination of the pteridine nucleus, *para* amino benzoic acid and glutamic acid. If the glutamic acid is replaced, the vitamin effect is also lost; on the other hand pteroic acid, both in combination with three molecules of glutamic acid (pteroyl triglutamic acid) and with seven glutamic acid molecules (pteroyl heptaglutamic acid) are biologically active.

It is stable to heat in neutral and alkaline solution, but unstable in acid solution. It is light sensitive.

Table 25 Content of folic acid in various foods.

	Folic acid µg/100 g
Calf liver	30–150
Beef or pork	1–5
Kidney	6–30
Eggs (each)	4
Potatoes	0–1·8
Green vegetables	9

SOURCES

Folic acid is present in all green-leaved vegetables and is also in liver and kidney (Table 25). Cooking may reduce the content considerably, and the availability from vegetable sources is not clear.

REQUIREMENTS

The minimum human adult requirement is believed to be about 0·1–0·2 mg. Daily recommended requirements have recently been established and are shown in Table 26.

Table 26 Daily requirements for folic acid
in humans expressed in μg/day.

		Folic acid $\mu g/day$
Adults		
Man		400
Woman		400
Pregnancy		800
Lactation		600
Children		
Both sexes	Under 1 year	50
	1–3 years	100
	4–6 years	200
	7–9 years	300
	10–12 years	400
Boys	13–15 years	400
	16–20 years	400
Girls	13–15 years	400
	16–20 years	400

Estimated requirements for animals are shown in Table 36 (page 194).

METABOLISM

No direct studies have been made of the absorption of folic acid. Apart from the limited quantities present in the liver no storage of this vitamin is known.

Many compounds, similar in chemical structure, interfere with the metabolic function of folic acid. Of these folic acid antagonists the most potent are those analogues which contain an amino group substituted for the hydroxyl group in position 4 of the pteridine nucleus. Aminopterin (4-amino folic acid) is the compound that has been studied most extensively. It appears to inhibit the conversion of folic acid to folinic acid. Aminopterin blocks the synthesis of nucleic acid in tissue cultures and the cells cannot complete their mitoses. Aminopterin has been used for the treatment of leukaemia, particularly in children.

PHYSIOLOGY

In 1948 a factor was discovered which was essential for the growth of *Leuconostoc citrovorum* and subsequently crystallized. This factor was named citrovorum factor, folinic acid or leucovorin.

In the liver folic acid is converted to folinic acid which is a tetrahydroderivative with a formyl group at position 5. This reaction is enhanced by ascorbic acid.

Except for the formylation of glutamic acid in the breakdown of histidine, however, the active form has the formyl group bound between positions 5 and 10 on tetrahydrofolic acid (Figure 36).

The function of folic acid is to act as a carrier of 'one carbon' moiety in an activated form for methylation reactions. This 'one carbon' moiety may be in the form of formyl (-CHO) formate (-COOH) or hydroxymethyl (-CH₂OH) which are metabolically interconvertible by an NADP dependent dehydrogenase (Figure 36).

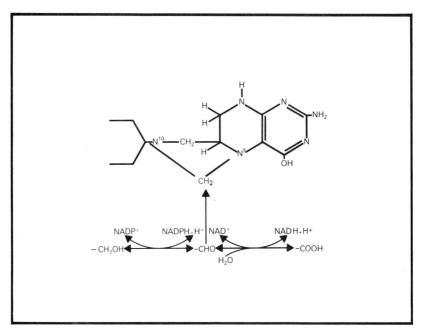

Figure 36 Interconvertibility of 'one carbon' moiety compounds and carriage of 'one carbon' fragment by folinic acid.

Sources of the carbon moiety are:
(a) Histidine via formimino glutamate.
(b) The beta carbon of serine.
(c) Glycine.
(d) Acetone and methanol.
Together with the methyl group of
 (i) Methionine.
 (ii) Choline by way of betaine.
 (iii) Thymine.
which are not carried direct by folic acid.
    The formyl carbon carried by tetrahydrafolic acid is used in many important reactions.
(a) As a source of carbons 2 and 8 in the purine nucleus.
(b) Conversion of glycine to serine.
(c) Methylation of homocysteine to methionine.

(d) Synthesis of thymine from uracil.
(e) Synthesis of choline.

These reactions are summarized in Figure 37. For some reactions specific methyl donors are utilized (e.g. methionine in choline synthesis). Vitamin B_{12} is also required in some of these reactions.

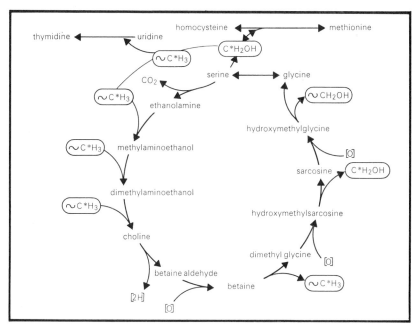

Figure 37 The role of folic acid and vitamin B in the formation of choline from dimethyl amino ethanol – i.e. for carriage of labile methyl group.

DEFICIENCY OF FOLIC ACID IN ANIMALS

Folic acid deficiency has been produced experimentally in many animal species. The constant finding is a macrocytic anaemia and leucopenia. The clinical picture of folic acid deficiency is determined by the results of disturbances of amino acid metabolism and of protein synthesis. Tissues which have a rapid rate of cell growth or of tissue regeneration, such as the epithelium of the gastrointestinal tract, the epidermis, and bone marrow, are particularly affected. A deficiency of folic acid results in a lowered hatchability of turkey eggs.

DEFICIENCY OF FOLIC ACID IN HUMANS

See also vitamin B_{12} (page 117).

The typical reaction to folic acid deficiency in the human is a megaloblastic red cell maturation in the bone marrow with a resulting macrocytic anaemia. This is accompanied by a leucopenia. (The appearances are similar to those seen in Plates 10 and 11).

Recent observations suggest that folic acid deficiency may present as a psychosis with mental deterioration. Folic acid deficiency can occur as a result of reduced dietary levels. This is seen most commonly in the tropics, but cases are also encountered in geriatric practice. There is usually a combination of impaired absorption and poor diet in these geriatric patients.

Intestinal malabsorption syndromes are also commonly accompanied by megaloblastic anaemia due to a folic-acid deficiency. The most common cause is steatorrhoea, but intestinal operations, particularly those producing 'blind loop' or a fistula between jejunum and colon, may also have the same effect.

A further cause of folic-acid deficiency is pregnancy. The developing foetus makes considerable demands on the maternal folic acid stores. If these are low at the beginning of pregnancy due to a poor diet, the stores become depleted and a megaloblastic anaemia occurs either near term or sometimes early in the puerperium. Megaloblastic anaemia in pregnancy occurs most commonly in the poorer sections of the community.

Megaloblastic anaemia due to a failure of folic acid function occasionally occurs in patients maintained for prolonged periods on certain anticonvulsants (phenytoin sodium and primidone). In this case the abnormality is probably an inhibition of the folic acid catalysis of nucleic acid formation.

THERAPY

Deficiency states

Folic acid in daily doses of 10 to 30 mg orally is adequate in most cases. Parenteral therapy with similar dosage is only rarely required. Maintenance therapy is sometimes necessary in sprue.

Folic acid should *not* be given as the sole therapy in Addisonian pernicious anaemia. It will produce a favourable haemopoietic effect initially, but it will neither relieve nor prevent degeneration in the nervous system; in fact it may precipitate it.

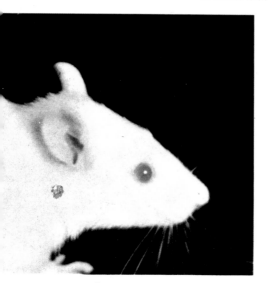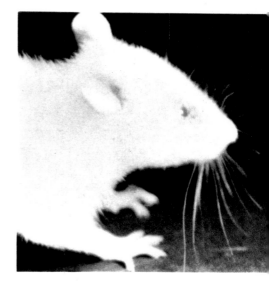

Plate 1 Vitamin A deficient rat (right) showing xerophthalmia compared with normal litter mate.

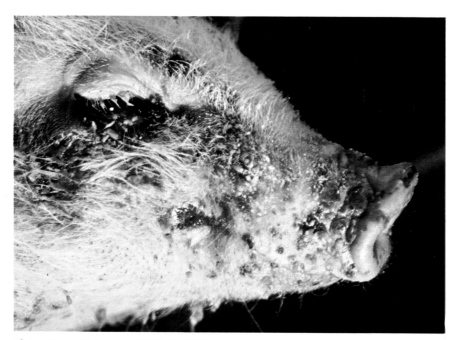

Plate 2 Dermatitis in a pig with biotin deficiency.

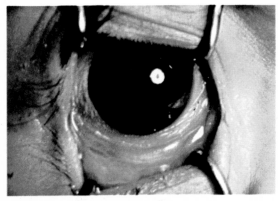

Plate 3 Xerosis. Note the hazy corrugated cornea, dry fatty conjunctival folds and Bitot's spot. Reproduced from *Assessment of Nutritional Status of a Community* by D. B. Jelliffe (1966) by permission of the World Health Organisation.

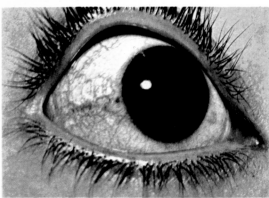

Plate 4 Example of typical Bitot's spots. Nine year-old Jordanian male. Serum vitamin A 4 μg/100 ml ('normal' 20–50 μg) liver vitamin A 21 μg/g fresh liver ('normal' above 45 μg). Excellent response to large doses of vitamin A. Reproduced by permission of Professor D. S. McLaren, Nutrition Research Laboratory, American University of Beirut.

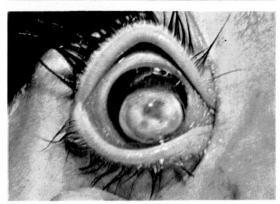

Plate 5 Keratomalacia. Fourteen month-old Jordanian male child. Serum vitamin A μg/100 ml ('normal' 20-25 μg) liver vitamin A 3 μg/g fresh liver ('normal' above 45 μg). By courtesy of Professor D. S. McLaren, Nutrition Research Laboratory, American University of Beirut.

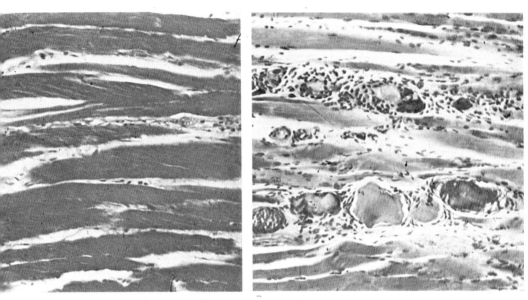

Plate 6 Muscle section in nutritional muscular dystrophy
(vitamin E deficiency) on right compared with normal.

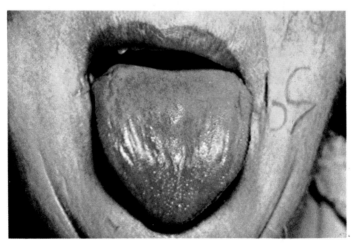

Plate 7 Typical tongue of nicotinic acid deficiency.
(Compare with normal tongue, Plate 12a.) Note the red,
raw, smooth appearance. By courtesy of Dr. Geoffrey
Taylor.

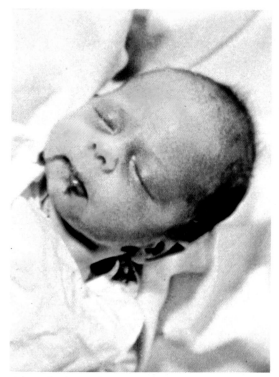

Plate 8 Blood-stained vomit in infant with haemorrhagic disease (vitamin K deficiency).

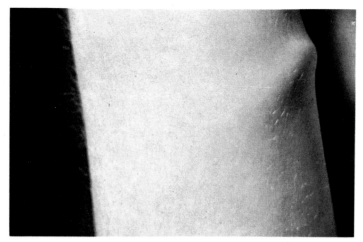

Plate 9 Myotactic irritability in an elderly patient with thiamine deficiency. By courtesy of Dr. Geoffrey Taylor.

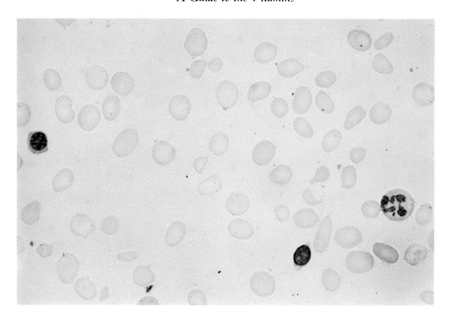

Plate 10 Typical blood picture in vitamin B_{12} deficiency. By courtesy of Prof. F. G. Hayhoe, Dept. of Medicine, University of Cambridge.

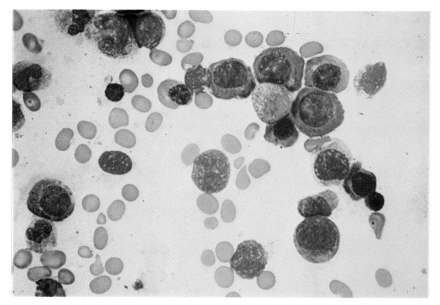

Plate 11 Megaloblastic bone marrow in vitamin B_{12} deficiency, patient whose blood is shown in Plate 10. By courtesy of Prof. F. G. Hayhoe, Dept. of Medicine, University of Cambridge.

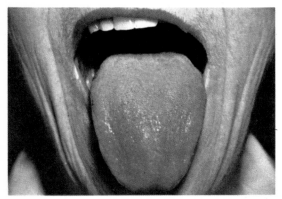

Plate 12
a. 'Normal' tongue.

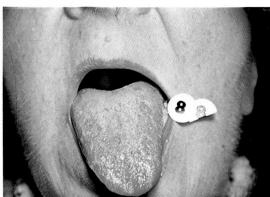

b. So-called 'geographical tongue' which many believe represents early B group deficiency probably involving riboflavine deficiency as a main component. Note the patchy shedding of filiform papillae, some fissuring, and fungiform papillae at tip.

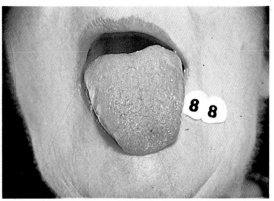

c. Same patient as (b) after 3 months' treatment with a high dose B complex preparation ('Becosym Forte'). By courtesy of Dr. Geoffrey Taylor.

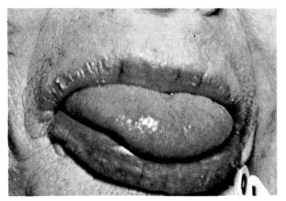

Plate 13 Riboflavine deficiency, showing angular stomatitis and severe cheilosis. Case seen in England 1966. By courtesy of Dr. Geoffrey Taylor.

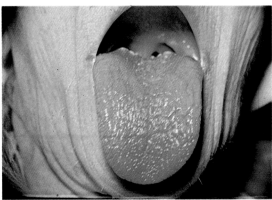

Plate 14 The typical tongue of a severe riboflavine deficiency. (England 1966.) (Compare with 'normal' in Plate 12a.) There is complete shedding of the filiform deep fissuring and marked fungiform papillae at tip. Angular stomatitis is also present. By courtesy of Dr. Geoffrey Taylor.

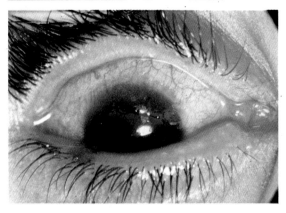

Plate 15 Vasculation of the cornea in riboflavine deficiency. Reproduced from *Assessment of Nutritional Status of a Community* by D. B. Jelliffe (1966) by permission of the World Health Organisation.

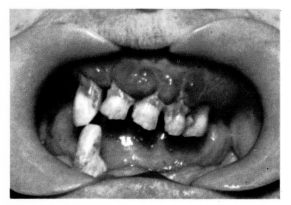

Plate 16 Swollen and bleeding gums in a middle-aged man with scurvy. Several of the teeth had become loose. By courtesy of Dr. Hansell, Westminster Hospital, London.

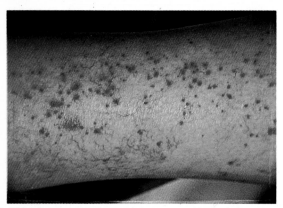

Plate 17 Skin petechiae in scurvy—photographed in England 1966. By courtesy of Dr. Geoffrey Taylor.

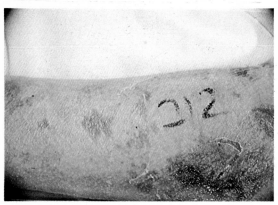

Plate 18 More extensive subcutaneous and intracutaneous haemorrhages in a case of scurvy. By courtesy of Dr. Geoffrey Taylor.

Vitamin B₁₂

Cyanocobalamin, Cobalamin (new terminology)
extrinsic factor (Castle), animal protein factor

In 1926 Minot and Murphy introduced the oral use of raw liver in the treatment of pernicious anaemia. From 1929 onwards Castle, from a series of studies, postulated that haemopoietic factor was formed from the interaction of a dietary (extrinsic) factor and a gastric (intrinsic) factor and was stored in the liver.

Progress in fractionation culminated in the isolation from liver of a red crystalline compound, vitamin B_{12}. It was subsequently shown that vitamin B_{12} as well as being the haemopoietic factor in liver also fulfilled the role of Castle's extrinsic factor. A tentative structure was first proposed in 1955 for the compound which was originally isolated – cyanocobalamin.

CHEMISTRY

Vitamin B_{12} is a red crystalline hygroscopic substance, freely soluble in water and alcohol but insoluble in acetone, chloroform or ether. It is labile in strong acid, alkali and light. The formula for cyanocobalamin is shown. The central ring structure is a 'corrin' ring system and bears a relationship to the porphyrins, but with a central cobalt atom. The cyano group can be replaced by acid groups or hydroxyl groups to give the cobalamins, nitritocobalamin and hydroxycobalamin, which are haemopoietically active. In its natural form vitamin B_{12} is probably bound to peptides or protein. Other analogues exist in nature that show activity in bacteria but not to higher animals

Crystalline cyanocobalamin and its aqueous solutions are stable at room temperature if they are not exposed to ultraviolet rays or intensive visible light. Vitamin C can attack it. Even vitamin B_1 or rather its decomposition products impair the stability of cyanocobalamin, the presence of nicotinamide intensifying the situation. In the production of multi-vitamin preparations, special protective measures are therefore necessary.

SOURCES

The amounts of vitamin B_{12} in food are very small. The main dietary sources are food of animal origin and their content is shown in Table 27. The vitamin is entirely or almost entirely absent from higher plants.

Table 27 Content of Vitamin B_{12} in various foods.

	Vitamin B_{12} $\mu g/100\ g$
Beef (lean)	2–3
Ox kidney	30
Ox liver	60
Pigs' hearts	25
Herrings	14
Mackerel	5
Cod and shellfish	0·5–0·8
Cows milk	0·3–0·6
Cheese	0·2–2
Eggs (each)	0·4

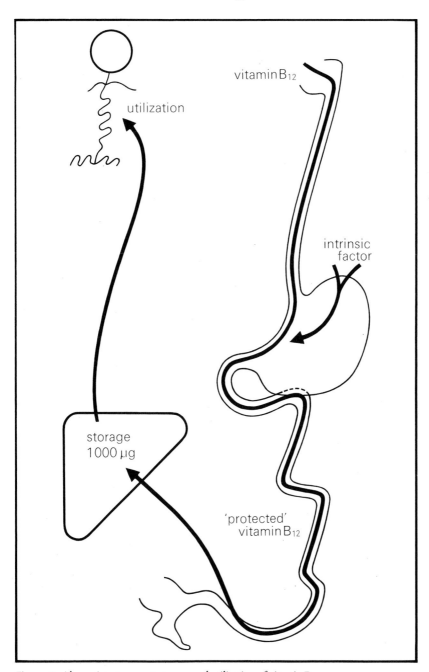

Figure 38 Absorption, transport, storage and utilization of vitamin B$_{12}$.

REQUIREMENTS

Vitamin B_{12} is synthesized in large quantities by the intestinal flora, particularly in ruminants. It is still not clear how much of this can be absorbed.

The exact amount of vitamin B_{12} required by the normal human is not known. According to the most recent evidence the minimum daily requirement for the vitamin has been set at less than 1 μg per day with a recommended daily allowance of 3 μg. For pregnant and lactating women 4 μg/day is recommended. For infants the level has been set at 0·3 μg/day, but further evidence is desirable for all these recommendations. Estimated requirements for animals are shown on Table 36 (page 194).

METABOLISM

The absorption of vitamin B_{12} from the gastrointestinal tract is dependent on a constituent of the gastric juice designated 'intrinsic factor' by Castle. The intrinsic factor is a constituent of gastric mucoprotein which is found in the cardia and fundus but not in the pylorus.

Recent work suggests that the intrinsic factor interacts with the vitamin B_{12} in the presence of calcium ions and protects it during its transit to the ileum.

Absorption of vitamin B_{12} takes place only in the ileum. There a highly specific binding site removes vitamin B_{12} from intrinsic factors in the presence of calcium and allows the vitamin to enter the mucosal cell for absorption. The percentage absorption is higher with smaller than with larger doses. The absorbed vitamin B_{12} is stored in the liver (Figure 38). Vitamin B_{12} is carried by at least two proteins (transcobalamin I, II) in the blood stream, the latter being physiologically more important.

PHYSIOLOGY

The physiological activities of vitamin B_{12} and of folic acid (see page 113) are interrelated but the exact mode of action of vitamin B_{12} and of its interaction with folic acid is still poorly understood.

It may act by cycling 5-methyltetrahydrofolate back into the folate pool, i.e. in the synthesis of folate polyglutamate, the active intracellular co-enzyme form. In this way, together with folic acid, it participates in the biosynthesis of labile methyl groups (Figure 36).

The formation of the labile methyl groups is necessary for the biosynthesis of the purine and pyrimidine bases which represent essential constituents of the nucleic acids. Disorders of nucleic acid synthesis in vitamin B_{12} deficiency are connected with this. The metabolism of labile methyl groups plays a significant part in the biosynthesis of methionine from homocysteine and choline from dimethylaminoethanol (Figure 37).

Methionine functions

(a) as an indispensable constituent of proteins,

(b) as a donor of methyl groups for the biosynthesis of the lipotropically active choline,

(c) for the formation of creatine which, after conversion to creatine phosphate, acts as an energy reserve maintaining ATP level in muscle tissue.

In all these reactions of the labile methyl groups folic acid plays an integral part too (see that section).

Another important function of vitamin B_{12} in intermediary metabolism is keeping the sulph-hydryl groups of enzymes in a reduced state. The reduced activity of glyceraldehyde-3-phosphate dehydrogenase which needs glutathione as a co-enzyme, is possibly responsible for carbohydrate metabolism being impaired in a vitamin B_{12} deficiency. Vitamin B_{12} also influences lipid metabolism via its effect on the thiols. A deficiency of this vitamin also results in a loss of the activity of the methyl malonyl coenzyme A isomerase. This enzyme converts the methyl malonyl co-enzyme A, which is derived from propionyl co-enzyme A by carboxylation, to succinyl co-enzyme A. In this reaction vitamin B_{12} probably acts as co-enzyme B_{12}. Co-enzyme B_{12} is distinguished by the fact that the cyano group of vitamin B_{12} is replaced by an adenine nucleoside. Much of the vitamin B_{12} in the organism seems to exist in this co-enzyme form.

Thus the fundamental role of the vitamin in metabolic processes is not limited to the haemopoietic system but occurs throughout the body. Part of the evidence for this is the great feeling of well being that occurs in the early stage of treatment of pernicious anaemia, even preceding changes in the red cells.

DEFICIENCY OF VITAMIN B_{12} IN ANIMALS

Most young animals show retarded growth on a purely vegetable diet or on a mixed diet containing alcohol extracted casein. This can be cured by the administration of vitamin B_{12}.

Nervous disorders occur in the pig; increased excitability, unco-ordinated movement and tender hind legs. The coat becomes rough and occasionally a local dermatitis develops. The thymus, spleen and suprarenals become atrophied, while the liver and tongue are frequently enlarged as a result of proliferation of granulomatous tissue. A microcytic anaemia is typical. (Diarrhoea and vomiting are occasionally observed in the case of young pigs.)

Halted growth and nervous disorders such as inco-ordination and ataxia also occur in calves which are fed with milk free of vitamin B_{12}.

Growth of poultry is halted without adequate B_{12} and mortality is high. Hatchability of incubated eggs may be severely reduced if the breeders' diet contained inadequate vitamin B_{12}. 'Dead-in-shell', under such conditions, show considerable embryonic malformations with maximum mortality around the 17th day of incubation.

If rats are given a diet free of B_{12} for several generations, the mortality rate in the young animals rises sharply and the weight of the animals at four weeks is reduced. The newborn of mothers who are on a vitamin B_{12}

deficient diet are often hydrocephalic and a great percentage show changes in the eyes such as distortion of the lens.

DEFICIENCY OF VITAMIN B_{12} IN HUMANS

Vitamin B_{12} deficiency may occur as a result of one or more of the following conditions: (Figure 38)

1 An inadequate dietary intake of vitamin B_{12}. This is rare for the vitamin is widely distributed but an occasional case is seen in geriatric patients and in strict vegetarians and rarely in tropical macrocytic anaemia.

2 A deficiency of the intrinsic factor. This may be due to deranged stomach activity as in Addisonian pernicious anaemia or follows total gastrectomy.

3 Bacterial or parasitic interference with the normal absorption of vitamin B_{12} in the alimentary canal (as in certain infections).

4 Defects in the capacity of the intestinal wall to absorb vitamin B_{12} (as in some cases of steatorrhoea).

The typical reaction to each of these deficiencies is the occurrence of a macrocytic anaemia. The erythrocytes are larger than normal, show great variation in size and a normal haemoglobin saturation (Plate 10).

The bone marrow shows a megaloblastic pattern of red cell maturation (Plate 11) as opposed to the usual normoblast pattern. The precursor cells of the megaloblastic series contain ribonucleic acid (RNA) and deoxyribonucleic acid (DNA) in greater amounts than normal and an increase in the RNA/DNA ratio.

Vitamin B_{12} is specifically indicated only for the treatment of Addisonian pernicious anaemia. In the other megaloblastic anaemias, folic acid is either more rapidly effective (e.g. nutritional macrocytic anaemia, sprue) or effective where B_{12} does not produce a response (e.g. megaloblastic anaemia of infancy or pregnancy). In these other macrocytic anaemias folic acid and vitamin B_{12} are often given simultaneously with advantage.

In advanced cases of Addisonian pernicious anaemia demyelination of the white fibres of the spinal cord occurs affecting the dorsal columns and the lateral columns (subacute combined degeneration of the cord) (Figure 39). In addition to subacute combined degeneration of the cord, hypovitaminosis B_{12} may give rise to a severe psychosis with extensive mental deterioration. Some patients have been described in whom this has occurred without the typical blood changes. Clinically the administration of either folic acid or vitamin B_{12} will produce:

1 Change from megaloblast to normoblast red cell maturation. This may be temporary with folic acid.

2 A subsequent reticulocyte rise, the extent of which is inversely related to the red cell count before treatment.

3 A rise in the red cell count to within normal limits.

However, although both folic acid and vitamin B_{12} will relieve the anaemia, only B_{12} will protect against or cure the spinal cord degeneration. It is believed that the latter finding is due to an interaction of folic acid and

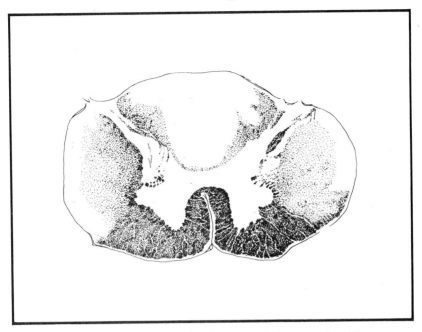

Figure 39 Transverse section of the spinal cord in a case of subacute combined degeneration of the cord.

B$_{12}$ in haematopoiesis so that less is available for activity within the spinal cord. Administration of folic acid alone, in Addisonian pernicious anaemia may precipitate subacute combined degeneration of the cord and its administration is contraindicated unless adequate doses of B$_{12}$ are given at the same time.

THERAPY

Deficiency states

During the stage of relapse of pernicious anaemia intramuscular doses of vitamin B$_{12}$ at the rate of 15–30 μg/day should be given. The individual doses need not be given daily. Alternatively, vitamin B$_{12}$ has been given in very large doses by mouth, or by mouth with intrinsic factor but neither of these methods can be advised for the response is variable.

In the patient treated successfully with intramuscular vitamin B$_{12}$ the first response occurs within about two days of the start of treatment and consists of an intense feeling of well-being and increase in the appetite.

After recovery has occurred and the blood values have returned to normal maintenance requirements of approximately 1 μg/day may be given as intramuscular doses of 30 μg at monthly intervals.

Other disorders

The general 'tonic' effect of vitamin B_{12} during the early stages of treatment of pernicious anaemia has led to the administration of the vitamin orally as a tonic in patients not suffering from pernicious anaemia. There is, however, no conclusive evidence of its value for this purpose.

Pantothenic Acid

Vitamin B$_5$ (sometimes called Vitamin B$_3$)

$$HOH_2C-\underset{\underset{CH_3}{|}}{\overset{\overset{CH_3}{|}}{C}}-CHOH-CO-NH-CH_2-CH_2-CO_2H$$

The presence of a pellagra-like dermatitis in chicks on a restricted diet was first described by Ringrose *et al.* in 1931. In 1933 Williams *et al.* gave the name pantothenic acid to a yeast growth factor of unknown constitution. The identity of the antidermatitis factor in chicks with pantothenic acid was recognised in 1939 and the compound was isolated from liver in the same year. Discovery of its constitution and synthesis came in 1940.

CHEMISTRY

Pantothenic acid is optically active. Only the dextrarotatory form is effective as a vitamin.

The free acid is a pale yellow viscous oil, soluble in water and alcohol, insoluble in benzene and chloroform and unstable to acids, bases and heat. The corresponding alcohol (panthenol) is more easily absorbed, and is rapidly converted to the acid in the body.

Pantothenic acid is d(+)-a(-dihydroxy-β,β-dimethylbutyryl-β-alanine). The structural formula is shown at the beginning of the chapter.

SOURCES

Pantothenic acid in bound form occurs as its name implies, in all animal and plant tissues. Rich sources are yeast, with 20 mg/100 g, and liver 8 mg/100 g. The content of pantothenic acid in various food sources is shown in Table 28.

Table 28 Content of pantothenic acid in various foods.

	Pantothenic acid mg/100 g
Meat, beef	0·3
pork	0·5
Sea fish	0·2–1·0
Eggs (each)	1·08
Cows milk	0·4
Wheat flour, wholemeal	0·5
75% extraction	0·23
Potatoes	0·6
Peas	0·34
Beans	0·14
Orange juice	0·16

REQUIREMENTS

The average daily excretion by humans is 5–6 mg or less. Thus a reasonable value for the requirement would be 5–10 mg and it is seen that the diet is normally adequate. In rodents synthesis by intestinal bacteria is believed to occur.

Requirements for animals are shown in Table 36 (page 194).

METABOLISM

Pantothenic acid, its salts and the alcohol are absorbed from the intestinal tract, probably by diffusion. Within the tissues the pantothenic acid is converted to co-enzyme A (Co-acetylase) (Figure 40).

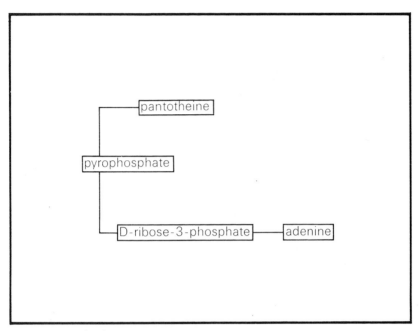

Figure 40 Formula of co-enzyme A.

Several substances, including salicylic and mandelic acid, have been reported to have an antagonistic action to pantothenic acid in micro-organisms. In animals certain analogues, including omega methyl pantothenic acid, can act as antagonists.

PHYSIOLOGY

The activity of pantothenic acid within the body depends on the activity of its conjugated nucleotide form – co-enzyme A. This co-enzyme is found in all tissues and is one of the most important co-enzymes for tissue metabolism.

The most important function of co-enzyme A is to act as a carrier mechanism for carboxylic acids. Such acids when bound to co-enzyme A have a high potential for transfer to other groups and such carboxylic acids are normally then referred to as 'active'. The most important of these reactions is the combination of co-enzyme A with acetate to form 'active acetate' with a high energy bond which renders the acetate capable of further chemical interactions, for example it is utilized directly by combination with oxaloacetic acid to form citric acid which enters the Krebs citric acid cycle. By this means 'acetate' derived from carbohydrates, fats or many of the amino acids can undergo further metabolic breakdown via the 'final common metabolic path' of the Krebs cycle. In the form of active acetate, acetic acid can also combine with choline to form acetylcholine, the chemical transmitter at the nerve synapse and can be used for detoxification of drugs including, for example, the sulphonamides.

Acetic acid in the form of active acetate is used as a precursor of cholesterol and thus also of the steroid hormones. Pantothenic acid deficiency produces profound effects in the adrenal gland with evidence of functional insufficiency. Co-enzyme A also has an essential function in lipid metabolism, fatty acids are activated by formation of the co-enzyme derivative and the removal of the acetate fragments in beta oxidation also uses another molecule of co-enzyme A. These active acetate fragments may directly enter the citric acid cycle or combine to form ketone bodies.

Decarboxylation of ketoglutaric acid in the citric acid cycle yields succinic acid which is then converted to the 'active' form by linkage with co-enzyme A. Active succinate and glycine are together involved in the first step of the biosynthesis of heme. Co-enzyme A thus plays a fundamental role in metabolism and particularly as a link between the various food products

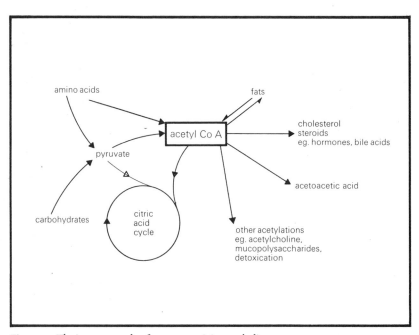

Figure 41 The important role of co-enzyme A in metabolism.

(carbohydrates, fats, and proteins) and their 'final common metabolic path'. This role is summarized in Figure 41.

The combination of carboxyl groups with co-enzyme A occurs at the terminal sulphydryl group. This high energy sulphur bond requires energy for its production derived from either ATP, another high energy sulphur bond, or an exothermic reaction (e.g. oxidative decarboxylation).

DEFICIENCY OF PANTOTHENIC ACID IN ANIMALS

Natural deficiency has been encountered in pigs who typically show a high-stepping action with their hind legs ('goose-stepping'), often accompanied by a scabby dermatitis around the eyes and snout. Experimental pantothenic acid deficiencies have been induced in most animal species.

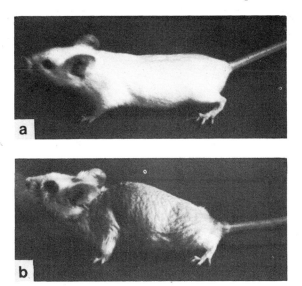

Figure 42 Dermatological manifestation of pantothenic acid deficiency (b) compared with a normal mouse (a).

Alopecia after loss of hair pigment (greying) is an early sign and in severe cases cutaneous ulceration may occur (Figure 42). Nervous system degeneration is frequently encountered with convulsions. A haemorrhagic exudative rhinitis progressing to a bronchopneumonia is a fairly common feature: while the alimentary canal shows intestinal distension, atrophy and ulceration. The liver frequently shows a fatty degeneration. The adrenal shows a haemorrhagic necrosis. A hypochromic anaemia is a constant feature probably due to poor heme synthesis in the absence of active succinate. Foetal resorption, abnormalities and sterility occur in some species. Bone changes and corneal vascularization have also been described.

DEFICIENCY OF PANTOTHENIC ACID IN HUMANS

Human pantothenic acid deficiency has been produced in volunteers by feeding a pantothenic acid deficient synthetic diet, or more rapidly by also including an antagonist in the diet. A deficient diet alone required about 12 weeks to produce recognizable symptoms. These included headache, fatigue, impaired motor co-ordination, paraesthesia, muscle cramps and gastrointestinal disturbances.

Effects on the heart — tachycardia and orthostatic hypotension — were seen in some of the subjects. Endocrine effects were shown by an eosinopenia and increased sensitivity to the hypoglycaemic effect of insulin.

Low pantothenic acid blood levels were commonly seen with generalized deficiency states. With these multiple deficiencies it is often difficult to distinguish the specific features occasioned by each factor.

The 'Burning Feet' syndrome, observed amongst prisoners of war and malnourished subjects in the Far East, responded to pantothenic acid containing preparations and not to the other members of the B complex and probably represents a specific deficiency.

THERAPY

Deficiency states

Pantothenic acid, often in the form of the alcohol, has been used in the 'Burning Feet' syndrome.

Other disorders

Applied topically, good results have been claimed in the healing of bed sores and varicose ulcers. Pantothenic acid by mouth has been found helpful in the prevention of streptomycin toxicity.

Many studies have been undertaken with parenteral pantothenic acid (50–100 mg/day) in the prevention and treatment of paralytic ileus. The results are still equivocal, but the balance of the evidence probably favours its use.

Biotin

Vitamin H

The toxic properties of raw egg white were first observed by Bateman in 1916. Boas (1927) found that certain foods were protective; biotin was isolated as the protective factor, its constitution determined and synthesized between 1936 and 1943.

CHEMISTRY

The chemical structure of biotin is shown on the previous page. It is a cyclic derivative of urea with an attached thiophene ring. There are eight different isomers of which only one, the so called d-biotin, is found naturally and has vitamin activity.

It consists of fine colourless needles slightly soluble in cold water, more soluble in alcohol, but practically insoluble in organic solvents. It is stable to heat, and not decomposed by acids or alkalis.

SOURCES

Biotin is widely distributed in small concentrations in all animal and plant tissues. High values are found in yeasts, liver and kidney. The biotin content of various foodstuffs is shown in Table 29.

Table 29 Content of biotin in various foods.

	Biotin μg/100 g
Meat, beef	2·6–3·4
veal	2·0
pork	5·0
lamb	5·9
chicken	10·0
Sea fish	0·1–3·0
Cows milk	2–5
Cheese	1·8
Eggs (each)	12
Wheat flour, wholemeal	7–12
80% extraction	1·4–3·0
Rice, polished	4–6
Apples	0·9
Orange juice	0·5–1·5

REQUIREMENTS

It is difficult to obtain a quantitative requirement for biotin. Balance studies show a urinary excretion in excess of dietary intake and large quantities are synthesized in man by the intestinal bacteria. The total intake from all sources probably amounts to between 150–300 μg daily.

Requirements for animals are shown on Table 36 (page 194).

METABOLISM

Biotin appears to be absorbed well from the small intestine. All cells contain some biotin, with larger quantities in the liver and kidneys.

Raw egg white contains avidin, a protein which combines with biotin and acts as an antagonist. However it is destroyed when eggs are cooked. Certain derivatives of biotin can act as antimetabolites to the parent substance.

PHYSIOLOGY

Present knowledge attributes an important co-enzyme role to biotin in the intermediary metabolism of carbohydrates, proteins and fats. It takes part in numerous carboxylation reactions, the labile carboxy-biotin functioning as an active form of carbon dioxide. Biotin may be involved in the following reactions, although some of these occur only in the vegetable kingdom:

Carboxylation of pyruvic acid to form oxaloacetic acid (Wood-Werkmann reaction).

Conversion of propionic acid to succinic acid via methyl malonyl Co A.

Transcarboxylation in the catabolism of various amino acids, e.g. leucine, isoleucine.

Conversion of acetyl Co A to malonyl Co A in the formation of long chain fatty acids.

Possible formation of citrulline, an intermediary substance in the synthesis of urea from ornithine and CO_2.

Possible effects on animal purine and pyrimidine synthesis.

Formation of aspartic acid.

DEFICIENCY OF BIOTIN IN ANIMALS

Biotin deficiency states can be induced in animals by destroying the biotin-producing flora by intestinal chemotherapeutics or feeding anatagonist, e.g. egg white disease. Recent work has shown that turkeys are very susceptible to biotin deficiency. Young poults show impaired growth, dry and brittle feathers, dermatitis and perosis. Defective bone and cartilage formation lead to distortions and shortening of the metatarsal bones in growing turkeys.

A deficiency syndrome in pigs shows as a dermatitis (Plate 2) on the ears, neck, shoulder and tail, which eventually covers the entire body. Cracks appear on the hooves, both in the wall and on the sides.

Broiler and replacement chicks are susceptible to biotin deficiency, with retarded growth, poor appetite, dermatitis of the feet, and perosis; eggs from biotin-deficient birds show poor hatchability and embryonic malformations. The disorder known as 'fatty liver and kidney syndrome' (FLKS) which commonly affects young broiler or replacement layer chicks between 10 and 30 days old has now been shown to respond to increased dietary levels of biotin. The cause of FLKS has not yet been fully defined, but affected birds suddenly show symptoms of paralysis and lie down either on their breasts with their heads stretched forward, or on their sides with their heads bent over their backs.

Fur-bearing animals may suffer from eczema, hyperkeratosis (alopecia) and pruritus. Severe conditions in minks and foxes may lead to poor fur quality (Figure 43), thickened and scaling skin, with inflammation and exudations around the eyes, nose and mouth. Depigmentation may occur to the fur around the eyes leading to a condition known as 'spectacle eyes'. A characteristic undesirable odour may develop, and males may show symptoms known as 'wet belly'.

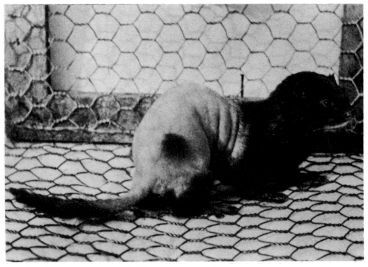

Figure 43 Fur loss due to biotin deficiency in mink fed on raw egg white. (By courtesy of Dr. A. Helgebostad, Heggedal, Norway).

DEFICIENCY OF BIOTIN IN HUMANS

Except in infants, natural deficiency state is extremely rare if it is seen at all. Experimentally induced human deficiency shows a mild dermatitis which develops after about four weeks and which by the 7th to 8th week shows desquamative patches, particularly of the extremities, and a greyish, dry scaly appearance. Atrophy of lingual papillae occurs with nausea and loss of appetite. The subjects complain of muscular pains, hyperaesthesia and lassitude. An anaemia is a fairly constant finding.

Two related conditions in infants, seborrhoeic dermatitis and desquamative erythroderma (Leiner's disease), are apparently connected with biotin deficiency since children suffering from these diseases have subnormal levels of biotin in blood and urine and respond to treatment with the vitamin.

THERAPY

Deficiency states

Administration of biotin, 5 mg daily by injection or 2–5 mg daily by mouth leads to spectacular improvement in the general condition of these infants within a few days and regression of the cutaneous lesions.

The vitamin appears to be of no value in other dermatological conditions.

Vitamin C

Ascorbic acid

Scurvy is one of the oldest diseases known to mankind. There is evidence of its existence in the Old Testament, in the Ebers papyrus and in the writings of Pliny. An early account of scurvy is that by Le Sieur de Joinville in the account of the crusade of St. Louis in Egypt in 1620. A knowledge of the curative value of vegetables must date back a very long time, for the American Indians have known for at least four centuries that scurvy could be cured by an infusion of spruce or pine needles.

In the Middle Ages scurvy was endemic in Northern Europe during the late winter months, because at that period the foodstuffs which nowadays provide the chief source of vitamin C (green and root vegetables) had not been introduced.

There are numerous sixteenth- and seventeenth-century writings on scurvy and, during this period, there seems to have been a tendency to associate scurvy and venereal disease. Mercury was used as a treatment, with disastrous results, and Felix Plater of Basle wrote that he believed that scurvy, like syphilis, had been brought from abroad by sailors!

By the end of the seventeenth century the new types of vegetables were available, and scurvy on land had become much less prevalent. By this time, however, it had become a formidable problem at sea with the longer voyages (see Figure 1). It is Dr. James Lind, Physician to the Fleet, who must be given the greatest credit for overcoming the problem. He was not in fact the first to discover the cure or prevention – Chatrier, Hawkins and Lancaster and perhaps others had recorded how scurvy might be controlled by a decoction of pine needles or citrus fruit. Their work had, however, been ignored and Lind rediscovered and increased the use of this therapy.

Lind's famous clinical experiment on scurvy, in which he showed that patients on lemon juice recovered while others treated at the same time but without lemon juice failed to do so, must be among the first examples of a controlled clinical trial and shows that these are not only confined to modern medicine. Lind indeed was responsible for the relief of both scurvy and typhus in the Fleet and probably helped as much as Nelson to break the power of Napoleon.

Over the past 150 years the further problems of this disease have been solved. The identity of the curative substance was proved in 1932 and the constitution of ascorbic acid and its synthesis accomplished during the next two years.

CHEMISTRY

Various substances have vitamin C activity in the body; the most important by far of these is l-ascorbic acid which is often equated with vitamin C for the sake of brevity.

Ascorbic acid is the enolic form of 3-keto-1-gulofuranolactone and has the structural formula shown at the beginning of the chapter. The d-isomer is devoid of activity. The endiol groups at the second and third carbon atoms are sensitive to oxidation and can easily convert into a diketo group.

The resultant dehydro-1-ascorbic acid is just as effective against scurvy as the reduced substance.

Ascorbic acid crystallizes out of water as square or oblong colourless crystals, slightly soluble in acetone, and the lower alcohols. A 0·5 per cent solution of ascorbic acid in water is strongly acid with a pH of 3.

Crystallized ascorbic acid is stable in air but in an aqueous solution it is attacked by atmospheric oxygen and other oxidizing agents. The resultant dehydroascorbic acid is oxidized further both rapidly and irreversibly; traces of heavy metal ions, for example, ions of copper, act as catalysts.

SOURCES

Ascorbic acid is widely distributed in high concentrations, particularly in citrus fruits and green vegetables. It is only found in the soft parts and not in the dry seeds. The average values expressed in mg/100 g for common foodstuffs are given in Table 30.

Table 30 Content of ascorbic acid in various foods.

	Ascorbic acid mg/100 g
Meat, beef and pork	up to 2
Liver, kidney	10–40
Cows milk	1–2
Potatoes	10–30
Cabbage	30–90
Brussels sprouts	90–150
Cauliflower	50
Broccoli	90–120
Carrots	9
Peas	14–32
Beans	10–20
Spinach	90
Tomatoes	20–33
Haws	160–800
Hips	1000
Peaches	5–25
Oranges, lemons	50
Grapefruit	40

The content of vitamin C is not only very uneven from one foodstuff to another, but also within one type, there are great variations according to species, degree of ripeness and provenance.

REQUIREMENTS

Unlike most species of animals the human body is unable to synthesize ascorbic acid. The human requirements are given in Table 31. The minimum per day is estimated at 0·4 to 0·5 mg per kg body weight equivalent to 25–30

Table 31 Daily requirements for ascorbic acid in humans expressed in mg/day.

		Ascorbic acid mg/day
Adults		
Man	Active	45
Woman	Active	45
	Pregnancy	60
	Lactation	80
Children		
Both sexes	Under 1 year	35
	1–3 years	40
	4–6 years	45
	7–9 years	45
	10–12 years	45
Boys	13–15 years	45
	16–20 years	45
Girls	13–15 years	45
	16–20 years	45

mg daily for the average adult. Some dispute still exists about the optimum intake for the human based on different criteria for normality. 45 mg/day will maintain an adequate body pool. In pregnancy and lactation higher doses are desirable (60 mg and 80 mg).

Requirements for animals are shown on Table 36 (page 194).

METABOLISM

The majority of animals are capable of synthesizing ascorbic acid within the body. Only a few, including man and the primate, together with the guinea pig, are dependent on exogenous sources. Female guinea pigs show higher buffy coat levels than males.

It is readily absorbed from the intestinal tract. It has been found that absorption is reduced with achlorhydria. Depression of absorption in certain intestinal infections has been claimed.

Unlike the majority of the water soluble vitamins, it appears that limited stores of ascorbic acid are held in the body. Thus signs of scurvy do not appear for some weeks in human volunteers receiving no vitamin C. It occurs in all body fluids and tissues but high levels are found in the liver (30–100 mg) and suprarenals (100 mg/100 g). These high adrenal levels are depleted when the gland is stimulated by adrenocorticotrophic hormone or during stress conditions. It would thus appear that ascorbic acid plays a part in corticosteroid synthesis.

Ascorbic acid is excreted in urine, sweat and faeces. The faecal loss is minimal and even with large intakes only 6–10 mg daily is excreted in this way. The loss in sweat is probably also low. The main loss, however, occurs in the urine. The urinary excretion depends on the body stores, intake and renal function. There is a glomerular filtration with active tubular reabsorption limited by a maximal rate. The resulting plasma threshold value is just over $1·0$ mg/100 ml in most circumstances.

Ascorbic acid is readily oxidized to the dehydro form. Both forms are found in body fluid and are physiologically active in the tissues. The interaction may perform an important function as a redox system, probably in association with glutathione.

A principal end product of the catabolism of l-ascorbic acid in the human organism is oxalic acid which is excreted with the urine. Apart from this substance, smaller amounts of 2,3-diketo gulonic acid appear. In rats and guinea pigs, on the other hand, l-ascorbic acid is catabolized, primarily oxidatively, to carbon dioxide.

PHYSIOLOGY

The full biochemical function of ascorbic acid is still unknown, although isolated reactions in which it is involved have been studied, viz:

1 Metabolic oxidation of certain amino acids including tyrosine. In scorbutic infants p-hydroxyphenyl pyruvic acid and homogentisic acid are found in the urine indicating incomplete oxidation of tyrosine.

2 Conversion of folic acid to folinic acid (see page 113). It may also affect the ability of the body to store folic acid.

3 According to more recent work, vitamin C plays an essential part in the transmission of iron from the plasma protein transferring into the organ protein ferritin which aids the accumulation of iron in the bone marrow as well as in the spleen and liver. Ascorbic acid may also be important for iron absorption from the intestinal tract.

In more general terms, it is known that ascorbic acid is required for the elaboration of the intercellular cement substance, and hence for growth and tissue repair. In ascorbic acid deficiency wound healing is delayed.

Ascorbic acid also may have a stimulating effect on the phagocytic activity of the leucocytes, on the function of the reticuloendothelial system and the formation of antibodies. The impaired formation of the intercellular substances of supporting tissue in the case of a vitamin C deficiency may be connected with disorders in the hydroxylation of proline to hydroxyproline, an essential component of the collagen fibres. But here too, further investigations are necessary to explain the exact mechanism.

The activity of ascorbic acid relative to resistance to infections is thought to be related to an effect within the adrenal cortex. High levels of ascorbic acid are found in this organ and it is believed that the vitamin is concerned with the hydroxylation of steroid hormones. Recent experiments suggest that ascorbic acid reduces the blood cholesterol levels.

For some of these diverse effects it is currently suggested that there is a metabolic link between ascorbic acid and cyclic AMP and cyclic GMP.

DEFICIENCY OF ASCORBIC ACID IN ANIMALS

Experimental ascorbic acid deficiency is difficult to produce in most animal species due to their ability to synthesize it. In the scorbutic guinea pig there is a diminution of activity and muscle atrophy of the feet. Capillary fragility and deficient wound healing are also seen.

In most species (with the exception of the guinea pig, monkey and man), the synthesis of vitamin C in the organs covers the individual requirements of the healthy animal under normal conditions. An exception seems to be the newborn calf which should be given a supply of vitamin C. When there is increased physical strain through illness, unfavourable environmental conditions or particular demands on capacity, a state can be reached in which the synthesis of vitamin C no longer covers the individual requirement. This is suggested by numerous reports of positive effects resulting from administering vitamin C to various species of animals. Thus it was observed, for example, in piglets, that ascorbic acid increases growth and haemoglobin production and alleviates some of the effects of diarrhoea. In poultry there is better heat resistance, further laying output, increased resistance to breakage of egg-shells, increased seminal production in young cocks, increased resistance to infections, and a reduced requirement for group B vitamins.

DEFICIENCY OF ASCORBIC ACID IN HUMANS

Gross vitamin C deficiency results in scurvy, a disease characterized by multiple haemorrhages. In adults manifest scurvy is preceded as a rule by lassitude, weakness, irritability, vague muscle and joint pains, and loss of weight. Bleeding gums, gingivitis and loosening of the teeth are usually the earliest objective signs (Plate 16). It must of course be appreciated that these early signs are absent in edentulous patients and this forms a trap for the unwary in geriatric practice. These are followed by minute haemorrhages under the skin (Plate 17), the site usually being determined by stress or trauma. Larger haemorrhages also occur (Plate 18). Large muscle haemorrhages are common, particularly in the thigh muscles. Peri-follicular congestion is frequent. In severe cases there may be haemorrhage into the conjunctivae, retina or cerebrum, or there may be bleeding from the nose, the gastrointestinal or genito-urinary tract.

In severe cases a typical haemorrhagic lesion occurs into the rib costochondral junction and neighbouring sub periosteal region. Rounded swellings appear in these regions. Infantile scurvy, which is usually due to lack of vitamin C in artificial feeds, generally occurs between the age of six months and eighteen months. As a rule it is first noticed that the infant cries on being handled, is irritable and loses appetite and weight. Tenderness of the extremities and pain on movement are almost invariably present. Haemorrhages may occur anywhere in the body, the commonest sites being under the periosteum of the long bones, in the gums, the skin, and the mucous membranes. Enlargement of the costo-chondral junction (the scorbutic rosary) is said to occur in about 75 per cent of scorbutic infants. Radiological changes in the long bones indicating a cessation of osteogenesis are a valuable aid to diagnosis.

THERAPY

Deficiency states

Ascorbic acid is specific in the treatment of scurvy. The dosage required can probably be assessed best by determination of the urinary excretion after saturation doses (see page 171). Depending on the speed at which saturation is required daily dosage varies between 200 and 2,000 mg.

Other disorders

In addition to its use in frank scurvy, there is an immense medical opinion favouring its use as an aid to the progress of recovery from a number of diseases. These findings are not supported by extensive controlled experiments, but nevertheless, the use of ascorbic acid in many of these conditions appears logical and justifiable. It does seem in fact that there is a great need to determine the significance of vitamin C depletion and saturation on the adrenal cortical function.

Anaemia and haemorrhagic disorders

The association of anaemia with scurvy has long been recognized. The value of the vitamin as an adjunct to iron therapy in nutritional anaemias is stressed.

In those patients with haemorrhagic disorders, showing laboratory evidence of increased capillary fragility, ascorbic acid should be given as a proportion respond dramatically.

Infectious diseases

Controlled studies have shown that in the course of infectious diseases the level of ascorbic acid in the system becomes very low whilst at the same time only small amounts are excreted. Especially noticeable is the vitamin C deficiency in active tuberculosis; it has been found to be proportional to the severity of the disease. In advanced cases maintenance of the ascorbic acid level at near 'saturation' point is recommended.

The value of large doses of vitamin C (1 g daily) in alleviating the signs of and hastening recovery from the common cold is still in doubt. Many doctors (including the author) feel justified in using it regularly for themselves and their families!

Gastrointestinal disturbances

In such conditions vitamin C deficiency may arise through impaired absorption, and parenteral treatment is indicated. The beneficial effect of vitamin C upon wound healing makes it essential that adequate amounts be administered in all cases of gastric and duodenal ulcer, especially as 'ulcer diets' are usually deficient in the vitamin.

Surgery and fractures

Histological investigations have shown that a deficiency adversely affects the formation of reticulum and collagen, thus delaying or preventing healing. Other studies have shown that there is greatly increased utilization of the vitamin in cases of trauma and in severe surgical cases.

Vitamin C is essential for the formation of bone and cartilage and for the formation of callus in the union of fractured bones. Fractures heal badly in a subject deficient in this vitamin.

Dental and oral conditions

Ascorbic acid given orally before and after dental extraction has been shown to result in rapid healing of the gum tissue together with rapid absorption of the alveolar bone margins. The prominence of such signs as spongy and bleeding gums and loosened teeth in scorbutic patients has led to the employment of vitamin C in similar lesions of the mouth in the absence of definite clinical signs of scurvy.

Infant feeding

Administration of the vitamin is essential to artifically fed babies since cow's milk and dried milk are not dependable sources of the vitamin. The synthetic substance is well tolerated by infants and its use is indicated when fresh fruit juices are disliked or cause gastric disturbances.

In psychiatry

High utilization rates for ascorbic acid have been found in many psychiatric patients and an improved mental state has been found in controlled trials with high doses of vitamin C.

Choline

$$\underset{H_3C}{\overset{CH_3}{\underset{H_3C}{|}}} \overset{+}{N} - CH_2 - CH_2OH$$

OH⁻

This compound is an accessory food substance which is now usually included in the vitamins. Choline can be synthesized in the liver. Nevertheless a dietary requirement can be demonstrated experimentally for many animal species.

Choline is a strong organic base which is widely distributed in nature either in certain phospholipids or as acetylcholine. The nutritional importance of choline was discovered in 1932.

It is a colourless crystalline structure which is remarkably hygroscopic. High levels (100–600 mg/100 g) are present in most animal tissues. Egg yolk is by far the richest source (up to 1,700 mg/100 g) and smaller quantities (up to 100 mg/100 g) are present in cereals and vegetables.

The normal daily intake of choline in adults on a mixed diet amounts to 300–1,000 mg. The urinary excretion in man amounts to about 5–9 mg/day and the estimated requirement is therefore probably about 10 mg/day, mainly by biosynthesis. Most of the dietary choline is broken down by intestinal bacteria into trimethylamine.

Requirements for animals are shown on Table 36 (page 194).

When labile methyl compounds (e.g. betaine and methionine) are present in adequate amounts choline may be synthesized in the body in quantities sufficient for normal needs.

Choline has several important biochemical functions within the animal body:

It can be converted in the body to betaine, which is a methyl donor for many transmethylation reactions.

It can be acetylated to form acetylcholine, the mediator of synaptic transmission.

It can prevent the accumulation of abnormal quantities of fat in the liver (lipotropic activity).

It probably acts by increasing phospholipid production.

In many animal species (e.g. dogs, rats, mice, hamsters, guinea pigs, rabbits, calves, pigs, ducklings and monkeys) choline deficiency with high carbohydrate diet, leads to the development of fatty liver. If the young animals survive the acute state a cirrhosis develops later.

In young rats choline deficiency also produces haemorrhagic degeneration of the kidneys and haemorrhages into many organs. In chicks and young turkeys a defect of the tibiotarsal joint is seen.

Because of the animal findings, choline has been incorporated in many 'liver protective' dietary supplements, but no evidence of a deficiency has yet been found for humans, although good results have been claimed in some countries following the use of such dietary supplements.

Part three

Technical Aspects

Vitamin
Assays

The original vitamin assays were based upon the determination of the specific effects of the vitamins in deficient animals and could be divided into curative and protective types. These techniques although determining the true availability of a vitamin in any substrate were nevertheless extremely expensive and time-consuming. In addition data from one species were not always relevant to those from another species.

Over the succeeding years attempts have been made to develop easier and more reliable methods of determination and these are now available for the majority of vitamins.

The methods in use at the present time can be divided broadly into four classes:

1 chemical
2 microbiological
3 animal curative and protective tests
4 biochemical

In any microbiological and biological assay procedure a comparison is made with known standards and the best techniques use a range of standards covering the unknown concentration.

PURPOSE OF VITAMIN ASSAYS

Assays and determination methods are needed for four main purposes.

Determination of the vitamin content of natural foods

These often present the greatest difficulty and are the least accurate. Interfering substances require complicated purification methods and the availability of the vitamin for absorption and utilization must be considered. In general terms older published figures markedly over-estimate the available vitamin content of foods. If losses in processing are also considered, recent work suggests that errors in some of the published figures amount to an overstatement by factors of up to ten to one. This aspect is considered in more detail on pages 177 to 186.

Vitamin content of pharmaceutical preparations

This is usually the most simple and accurate group. Not only are the vitamins usually present in a pure and unbound form, but the exact nature of other substances is known. Modern methods usually give good reliable results for pharmaceutical preparations.

Total content of vitamins in supplemented food and feeding stuffs

The estimation of the added vitamin is usually reasonably reliable although substances originally present in the food may interfere with the methods that are employed. Total content, however, is open to the same objections as those for natural foods.

Vitamin levels in biological fluids and tissues

Two problems exist in biological materials: the rather low content per unit volume in the majority of fluids and tissues and the presence of other substances which render accurate estimation difficult.

ASSAY METHODS FOR VITAMINS

Details of the assay methods are not considered in this book for they are available in the standard analytical reference books. Principles of the methods used for each vitamin and a note on the accuracy of the estimations is considered relevant.

Vitamin A

Vitamin A can be estimated by colour reaction, by ultraviolet absorption, and by animal assay techniques. For accurate determination preliminary chromatographic separation is desirable.

Fairly good estimates of the available vitamin A content of foods are obtained by existing analytical methods. Over-estimation may result, however, if effective purification steps are not included.

Calculation of the vitamin A activity derived from carotene over-estimates the true available vitamin A for some of the carotene is not in a form which can be converted. This is particularly true in the case of fresh vegetables. Estimates obtained after cooking are nearly always too high.

Vitamin D

The only method that can be used for complicated mixtures (including foods) is an animal assay. A U.V. absorption test and a fluorimetric estimation are only applicable after extraction of the vitamin D from simple mixtures usually by chromatographic separation.

Vitamin E

A colorimetric estimation is the one most frequently used but the reaction is non-specific and tocopherol must be separated out by chromatography first. Levels in biological fluid can be determined fluorimetrically. Animal tests are available but are now rarely used. In foods the available techniques still over-estimate the true levels and a more specific test is desirable.

Vitamin K

Vitamin K can be estimated by colorimetric or fluorimetric methods but these chemical methods are only appropriate for pharmaceutical preparations, if necessary after chromatographic separation. The only technique for food is a biological determination in animals, but the method is far from ideal.

Vitamin C

Vitamin C is normally determined either by oxidation-reduction processes or from characteristic colour reactions. The chemical conversions all depend on the endiol grouping and are not specific therefore for ascorbic acid. The most specific methods of determination are those where chromatographic separations are combined with any of the following methods:

(a) Tillmann's oxidimetric titration with 2,6-dichlorphenolindophenol is very popular. Other common oxidizing agents are iodine or chloramine solutions. The oxidizing process can also be carried out photometrically; here an excess of Tillmann's reagent, methylene blue, phosphotungstic acid or phosphomolibdino tungstic acid is used and the changes in the intensity of the colour are measured. The disadvantage of the oxidimetric processes is that they also estimate other substances with a similar redox potential to ascorbic acid. Dehydroascorbic acid can only be titrated after it has been reduced to ascorbic acid by hydrogen sulphide, cysteine, homocysteine or, rarely, a selective reduction by micro-organisms.

(b) The best known, non-oxidimetric processes are the photometric determination of the bis-2,4-dinitrophenyl hydrazone of dehydroascorbic acid, and the reaction with diazotized 4-methoxy-2-nitroaniline or with 2-nitroaniline. Here, after splitting the endiol group by the diazonium salt, the corresponding semi-hydrazide of oxalic acid is formed and the alkali salts of this are coloured.

(c) More specific than the above methods, although not quite so exact, is polarographic determination. Protective tests in guinea pigs have been described but are not now used. The different chemical tests, due to their non-specific nature give variable results on the same food. Moreover, they do not assess the biological availability of the ascorbic acid.

Vitamin B_1

Thiamine can be estimated fluorimetrically after conversion to thiochrome. The method is accurate but there is sometimes difficulty in liberating thiamine from its bound form.

Less used methods include a straight fluorimetric method, a polarographic method, a microbiological method involving various organisms and animal curative and protective tests. The only advantage of the microbiological test is that some organisms respond to free thiamine and some to thiamine pyrophosphate so that differential estimations are possible.

Vitamin B_2

Riboflavine can be estimated photometrically (particularly for example pharmaceutical preparations), fluorimetrically, polarographically, microbiologically and by an animal assay technique.

The main problem here is the assessment of the availability of riboflavine from the various natural sources. Biological methods are awkward to use but probably more accurate.

Vitamin B_6

The determination of pyridoxine in pharmaceutical preparations is usually carried out colorimetrically but polarographic and fluorimetric methods are also available. Unfortunately none of these is ideal for food determinations. Microbiological techniques are available which can estimate the individual member of the B_6 group but they are not suitable for routine use. An animal curative test has also been described but is now rarely used.

Nicotinic acid

A photometric method is the one normally employed. It is important to appreciate that nicotinic acid extractable by acid hydrolysis is the only one which is biologically available, and this technique should therefore be used for any assessment of the level available in the body.

In addition to this photometric method, polarographic, fluorimetric, microbiological and animal curative tests are available but not widely used.

Folic acid

In simple mixtures, e.g. pharmaceutical preparations, a direct photometric, fluorimetric or polarographic determination is possible.

Since there are no methods which can be applied to complex mixtures (e.g. food) the folic acid must first be released, then determined microbiologically. The specificity is not great and present techniques are inaccurate.

Vitamin B_{12}

In simple media vitamin B_{12} can be estimated photometrically. Microbiological assay tests are available but are non-specific, cumbersome and not easily applied to foods. The activity of extracts or derivatives can be determined from the reticulocyte response in pernicious anaemia patients.

Pantothenic acid

A microbiological method is normally used but this is not applicable to routine examination of food. At the moment no specific chemical method exists. An animal assay technique has been described.

Biotin

No accurate and reasonably simple method of estimation is yet available for biotin in food substances, the only satisfactory method involving hydrolysis, then microbiological determination. An animal assay method is available but rarely used.

Choline

The determination of choline is complicated by the various forms in which it may be present in the sample. Simple extraction with water or alcohol is sufficient to remove free choline, but more exacting procedures must be employed for the extraction of total choline. Microbiological, gravimetric, colorimetric and chromatographic methods have been employed to estimate the choline content of the extract.

Examination for Vitamin Nutritional Status in the Human

The diagnosis of a vitamin deficiency state presents no problem to the clinician when it is present in its classical and overt form. Many of the physical signs are specific to the individual vitamin deficiencies although most patients in practice show a mixed picture due to the deficiency of various nutritional factors. The main difficulty in the diagnosis of overt vitamin deficiency is the failure on the part of the physician to appreciate that such a deficiency may exist in the patient. In most industrialized countries the current but fallacious teaching is that vitamin deficiencies no longer occur.

However, attempts are being made to advance the diagnosis of the disease. In addition nutritionists have become interested in the possibility of a 'sub-clinical deficiency state'. This may be defined as a state in which the level of a vitamin in the tissues is low, but in which the classical symptoms and signs of the disorder are not present. Much work has been undertaken recently to determine whether such sub-clinical deficiency states do in fact produce any mild symptoms or signs (e.g. lassitude) or whether they have any causative role in other disorders.

The sequence of events which leads to a classical vitamin deficiency state is shown diagrammatically in Figure 44. The first stage is an inadequate intake of the vitamin into the body to meet the needs at that particular time. This can result not only from a primary dietary lack, but also from poor absorption, impaired transport or excessive requirements. When the intake is inadequate then tissue desaturation takes place. The rate at which this occurs is variable from one vitamin to another depending upon the stores.

Once tissue desaturation has reached a critical level then the metabolic function of the vitamin is lost and changes occur in specific enzyme activity. When these in turn reach a critical level the clinical picture of the vitamin deficiency disorder appears.

Obviously true vitamin deficiency can only be diagnosed in the presence of evidence of clinical disorder. Examination of the vitamin intake or of tissue desaturation of the vitamin can merely give evidence of vitamin levels below the optimum. In order to determine whether such levels have clinical significance it is important to make such examinations. Moreover they have a place in attempting specific diagnoses in patients in whom multiple deficiencies exist or who show a deficiency state superimposed on another disorder. At the present time vitamin deficiency can be determined by any of the following techniques:
1 Determination of dietary levels.
2 Estimation of tissue desaturation.
3 Measurement of specific enzyme activity depression.
4 Clinical examinations.

DETERMINATION OF THE VITAMIN CONTENT OF THE DIET

The subject is considered in detail on page 176. Problems exist for the estimation of the true absorbable vitamin content. These include inadequate data on the true vitamin content of the raw food, lack of knowledge of

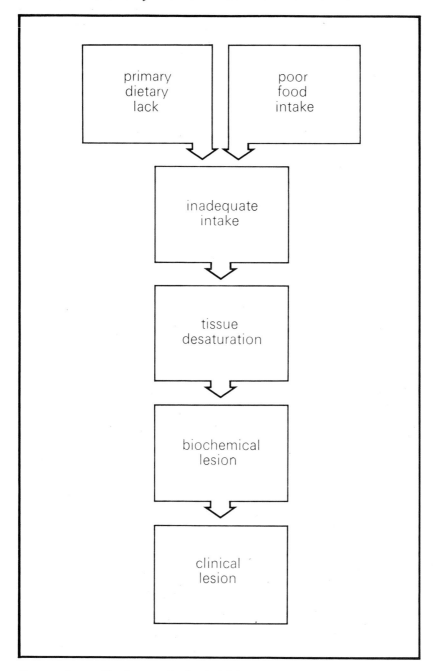

Figure 44 Stages of development of a vitamin deficiency.

the proportion of this original vitamin content which is capable of being absorbed from the intestinal tract and inadequate data on the losses during the processing of the food. Reliable estimates involve analysis of aliquots from the plate coupled with weighed portions.

Thus though determination of the vitamin intake from the food can be correlated with the findings of a vitamin deficiency within the body they should be used with caution as a diagnostic test for vitamin deficiency.

TESTS FOR TISSUE DESATURATION

Three types of test have been used to determine tissue desaturation. Two of these techniques are usually easy to perform but do not cover the entire problem. The third technique is usually complicated and is only suitable for research examinations. The problems which are encountered in the interpretation of tests of these three types can best be exemplified by the specific case of ascorbic acid for which all three methods are available. The methods used and the typical problems of interpretation are as follows:

Measurement of blood levels with or without a test dose

Sensitive and reasonably simple chemical techniques now exist for determination of the level of many vitamins in the plasma. However, the vitamin in the plasma is not filling a metabolic function, but is merely in transit from one tissue to another. Its lack might or might not indicate the status of intracellular vitamin levels.

A well nourished adult who is placed on a diet free of ascorbic acid shows a fall in the serum ascorbic acid level almost to zero in about six weeks. Several more weeks' deprivation is, however, needed before the first signs of scurvy appear. Thus while it is true that all patients with scurvy will have very low plasma ascorbic acid levels the converse is not true and low plasma levels can be found in the absence of any clinical evidence of ascorbic acid deficiency. In view of the low levels of most of the vitamins in blood and tissues chemical determination is often difficult. To overcome this problem a 'loading dose' of the vitamin is given.

Determination of the plasma level after a loading dose in general reflects the proportion of the vitamin dose which has been taken into stores or tissues. It is, however, difficult to make the technique completely quantitative. If high doses of the vitamin are given, the plasma level rises above the renal threshold and loss occurs in the urine.

Measurement of the renal excretion rate with or without a test dose

While the urinary excretion of the vitamin per twenty-four hours usually correlates reasonably well with the prevailing dietary intake, it is not always a true reflection of the tissue state. This is true to a certain extent with ascorbic acid, but is more obvious for vitamin A with its high tissue reserves. The same problems exist with this determination as with the plasma determination with or without a test load.

Moreover, there are problems in obtaining twenty-four-hour samples of urine in many circumstances in which assessment of the vitamin state is important. Use has been made of smaller samples and the levels are then correlated with creatinine excretion. Creatinine is used as an index because at normal plasma levels, it gives a reasonably simple and reliable measurement of the extent of direct filtration through the glomeruli. Random urine sample determination correlated with creatinine, although among the easiest to perform for mass survey purposes, gives the least valid and useful information.

Measurement of tissue levels

This is the only one of the three techniques which gives a true representation of vitamin desaturation. Measurement of tissue levels is often difficult to undertake due to problems of tissue sampling and in the analytical technique.

In the case of ascorbic acid two methods have been used for determinations of tissue ascorbic acid levels. In the first of these examination is made of the level in the buffy coat, consisting of leucocytes and platelets. This can be shown to correlate very well with the first signs of scurvy and is the recommended technique for ascorbic acid determinations. The actual determination is, however, rather laborious. Attempts have also been made to determine the degree of tissue saturation of ascorbic acid by an intradermal test using dichlorophenolindophenol. The method depends upon the presence in the skin of reducing substances and is therefore non-specific. In spite of this the results seem to correlate reasonably well with the dietary intake of the vitamin, but the technique suffers from the disadvantage of all such determinations which are non-specific.

All these techniques, however, seek to determine the level of saturation of the vitamin in the body and take no account of the metabolic needs. Thus they may show a deficiency but do not show whether this deficiency matters for the maintenance of normal tissue integrity.

TESTS FOR BIOCHEMICAL METABOLIC EFFICIENCY

The tests for biochemical metabolic efficiency attempt to determine the vitamin level in relation to that required by the tissue to maintain its integrity. They give a more reliable indication of the vitamin state relative to the vitamin need at the time. Unfortunately, however, such tests are only available for a very limited number of vitamins.

If this type of test is to be undertaken it is important to utilize a technique which is specific to the vitamin and in which alternative pathways for metabolism or alternative co-enzymes do not exist.

Even if specific biochemical lesions can be determined, the significance of these lesions for clinical disorders is not always clear. In most metabolic pathways there are only one or two rate-limiting steps. If the vitamin concerned does not take part in any of these rate-limiting steps then the finding of impaired metabolic efficiency in a step in which the vitamin takes part may have no direct significance in relation to the integrity of the metabolic process as a whole.

Typical examples of this type of test are the pyruvate determinations and T.P.P. effect for thiamine deficiency (page 172); the examination for creatinuria in tocopherol deficiency (page 170); study of tryptophan metabolism for pyridoxine deficiency (page 172); prothrombin estimation for vitamin K deficiency (page 170).

CLINICAL ASSESSMENT OF VITAMIN DEFICIENCY

Specific symptoms and signs exist for most of the vitamin deficiencies, and when they exist in their classical form these can be readily recognized. Recent experience in Great Britain has demonstrated that mild abnormalities which could fit in with a vitamin deficiency are seen not infrequently in certain sections of the population. Since the examination is by its very nature subjective there is often some doubt as to the significance of these clinical signs. Unfortunately only a very few objective methods of determining clinical features of vitamin deficiency exist (e.g. dark adaptation test for vitamin A deficiency).

As with any clinical examination it is important to take a full history and make a full physical examination before reaching a diagnosis.

Nevertheless, within this framework of a general history and physical examination, certain areas of the body will provide the greatest amount of information on vitamin deficiencies and attention should be particularly directed to these when poor nutrition is suspected. The areas concerned are the eyes, the skin and the mouth. A summary of the typical lesions seen in particular systems of the body as a result of vitamin deficiency is given in the following section. Details of the individual findings will be found in the appropriate sections in part II.

The skin

Deficiencies of the vitamins are often associated with alteration in skin and hair in experimental animals, and it was tempting for these animal findings to be translated into human diseases by physicians eager to treat difficult dermatological problems. As a consequence of such haphazard studies the literature abounds with contradictory statements. In more careful recent studies many of the previously reported observations have not been confirmed and in only a few lesions can a specific vitamin deficiency be established.

Vitamin A

Skin keratinisation (toad skin) was formerly attributed to a deficiency of vitamin A. Recent studies suggest deficiency of essential fatty acids to be a more likely cause.

Characteristic follicular lesions, hard and deeply pigmented with a central keratinized epithelial papule, have been described as being due to vitamin A deficiency. Confirmation is needed.

Signs of hypervitaminosis A may include a dry rough skin. High doses of carotene (provitamin A) can produce a yellowish discolouration of the skin which may be confused with jaundice.

Vitamin A has been used for a variety of skin disorders – specifically topical retinoic acid may be valuable in the treatment of keratoses and acne.

Vitamin K
Cutaneous purpura may reflect a prothrombin deficiency resulting from vitamin K deficiency.

Ascorbic acid
Ascorbic acid deficiency results in a characteristic loss of intercellular ground substance and a weakening of collagen supporting the capillary wall. Ascorbic acid is also concerned with the metabolism of the amino acids tyrosine and phenylalanine, precursors of skin melanin.

The typical skin reaction of scurvy is rather diffuse petechial haemorrhages (Plate 17). Hyperkeratotic follicular papules on the calves and buttocks with spiral and unerupted hairs have also been described.

Pyridoxine
Although the lesions of pyridoxine deficiency superficially resemble those of essential fatty acid deficiency, differences exist between the two conditions. In pyridoxine deficiency there is an atrophy of the epidermis, hair follicle and sebaceous glands with a loose hyperkeratosis.

The pure skin lesions characteristic of pyridoxine deficiency have been studied in man by the use of the pyridoxine antagonist 4-desoxypyridoxine. Seborrhoea-like·lesions were seen about the eyes, the nasolabial fold and mouth with extension to the eyebrow and behind the ear. The moist areas of the body showed an intertrigo. A scaly pigmented dermatitis occurred sometimes around the neck, forearms, elbows and thighs. However, the relationship of impairment of pyridoxine function to clinical seborrhoeic dermatitis has not been established.

Riboflavine
Riboflavine deficiency produces characteristic, but not constant, skin lesions. The variability may be related to local trauma. The typical lesions in man are cheilosis, angular stomatitis (Plates 12–15), nasolabial seborrhoea, and scrotal or vulval dermatitis.

Nicotinic acid
Nicotinic acid deficiency produces pellagra. The initial change is a temporary redness like that of sunburn. This clears spontaneously to reappear later as a more severe red macula reaction, which coalesces and forms a dark red or purplish eruption followed by desquamation. Areas of friction and exposure are most involved – face, neck, hands and feet. (Figures 34, 35). The area is often oedematous and ulceration sometimes occurs.

There is often a sharp margin to the hand lesion and it is often termed 'pellagrous glove'.

Pantothenic acid

Although pantothenic acid deficiency results in greying of the hair and ulcerations in animals, no similar associations have been proved for the human. War-time prisoners in the Far East suffered from the 'Burning feet' syndrome which appeared to be a true pantothenic acid deficiency. It is probably a symptom of a nerve lesion rather than a skin lesion. Some skin reactions resembling riboflavine deficiency have responded to pantothenic acid administration. Pantothenic alcohol is widely used as a constituent of skin applications in many countries.

Biotin

In the infant a biotin deficiency can produce a severe local desquamatory dermatitis.

The mouth

The classic descriptions of the vitamin B deficiencies affecting the mouth clearly distinguish between members of the B complex. Recent studies, however, suggest that it is difficult to distinguish between individual members of the B group, due to the fact that many deficiency states are due to lack of more than one vitamin.

Although strictly speaking referable to the skin the angles of the mouth and the lips are normally examined in relation to the mouth and are therefore considered in this section.

Riboflavine

Ariboflavinosis produces cheilosis and angular stomatitis with a sore tongue. The tongue is described as being magenta-coloured with deep fissuring and prominent papillae (Plate 14).

Nicotinic acid

Lack of this vitamin also produces gingivitis, stomatitis and a fiery glossitis, the tongue being swollen and beefy red (Plate 7).

Pyridoxine

Volunteers with impairment of pyridoxine function brought about by the administration of anti-vitamins show a cheilosis and glossitis. Recent work suggests that some of the lesions reputedly characteristic of ariboflavinosis may in fact be due to pyridoxine deficiency.

Vitamin B_{12}

Although characteristic anatomical lesions of the mouth have not been reported for vitamin B_{12} deficiency, many patients with pernicious anaemia complain of a sore tongue before treatment is commenced. This clears rapidly with administration of vitamin B_{12} and is probably related to the deficiency.

Ascorbic acid

Deficiency of ascorbic acid as seen in severe scurvy produces bleeding gums, gingivitis and a loosening of the teeth (Plate 16). In addition to this, petechial haemorrhages may be found in the mouth particularly in relation to rough teeth. In edentulous people it is more difficult to diagnose scurvy from mouth lesions.

Biotin
In infants atrophy of the lingual papillae has been reported in association with the characteristic dermatitis.

The intestinal tract

Thiamine
Thiamine deficiency can produce a diarrhoea with abdominal distension and colicky pains.

Nicotinic acid
Diarrhoea is an almost constant accompaniment of severe nicotinic acid deficiency.

Pantothenic acid
Naturally occurring pantothenic acid deficiency has not been described, but in volunteers rendered deficient, an intestinal atony has been produced. The finding of intestinal atony in animal deficiency and in experimental human deficiency first led to the trial of pantothenic acid in post operative paralytic ileus. Subsequent controlled trials have confirmed its therapeutic value in this condition.

The eye

Vitamin A
Vitamin A deficiency can produce characteristic lesions in both the retina and the anterior segment of the eye.

In the retina the characteristic symptom is poor dark adaptation due to a deficiency of rhodopsin in the rods. In the anterior segment the characteristic lesion of vitamin A deficiency is xerophthalmia. In mild cases this shows itself as a xerosis – largely represented by a dryness of the conjunctival sac (Plate 3). However, in more severe cases this can progress to keratomalacia with severe ulceration (Plate 5). In advanced and untreated cases it can lead to blindness. This disorder is one of the main causes of blindness in the world at the present time, particularly in tropical areas.

Riboflavine
A characteristic vascularization of the cornea is found not uncommonly in ariboflavinosis (Plate 15). Associated with this sign, patients may complain of conjunctivitis especially affecting the lower lid, a feeling of grittiness, lachrymation and failing vision.

In some other cases a corneal epithelial dystrophy has been described, which though probably associated with multiple vitamin B deficiency, may have been related to ariboflavinosis.

Thiamine

A widespread condition of nutritional amblyopia has been described. This is found in many tropical countries. The exact aetiology of this disorder is at present unknown, but there is evidence to suggest that a thiamine deficiency may be one of the important causes.

Although Wernicke's encephalopathy is a disorder of the central nervous system, it commonly manifests itself with ocular signs of which nystagmus, external rectus fatigue, and paralysis and loss of visual acuity are the most common findings.

Nicotinic acid

Nicotinic acid deficiency is also reputed to be a cause of nutritional amblyopia. Most deficiencies, however, involve several vitamins and there is no direct evidence associating nicotinic deficiency with the amblyopia.

Acute nicotinic acid deficiency can also produce an encephalopathy very similar to that found in acute thiamine deficiency. As with the thiamine deficiency, ocular symptoms may be present including bilateral nystagmus and complete ophthalmoplegia.

Ascorbic acid

Although the haemorrhagic signs in scurvy are normally found in other areas, intra-ocular haemorrhages have sometimes been the first presenting sign in this disease.

Vitamin K

One of the sites of a haemorrhage in haemorrhagic disease of the newborn has been the retina.

Hypervitaminosis D

In hypervitaminosis D there are deposits in the conjunctiva of clear crystal-like particles in the region of the palpebral fissure, while calcified sclera have also been demonstrated.

Hypervitaminosis A

Acute hypervitaminosis A can produce a marked rise in cerebro-spinal fluid pressure and papilloedema has been observed in some cases with accompanying visual disturbances. In chronic hypervitaminosis A extraocular muscle paralyses and occasionally exophthalmos have been found as well as papilloedema.

The central nervous system

Thiamine

Thiamine deficiency produces two effects within the central nervous system. Acute thiamine deficiency produces Wernicke's syndrome (cerebral beri-beri) with its gross mental changes. The picture is often complicated, for the encephalopathy usually develops when an acute thiamine lack is superimposed on the background of a chronic deficiency. In these acute cases the most important sign is mental confusion leading to coma; in the typical Wernicke's syndrome a bilateral sixth nerve paralysis is also found. In less severe forms of the disorder nystagmus is found but no true sixth nerve paralysis, and in some relatively mild cases there may only be a little mental confusion. The sixth nerve disorder responds rapidly to the administration of thiamine but the mental changes are far more difficult to reverse.

Korsakoff's psychosis, a confusion state with confabulation and poly-neuritis, has also been attributed to thiamine deficiency but the relationship is not clear.

In chronic thiamine deficiency the typical nervous system finding is a neuritis. In the early stage the sensory nerves are affected, but in the more prolonged deficiency, motor nerves are also involved, with muscle wasting and paralysis – typically wrist- and foot-drop.

Pyridoxine
Pyridoxine deficiency produced by administration of an antagonist in vol-unteers sometimes produces a peripheral neuritis. Patients treated clinically with certain drugs (including isoniazid and penicillamine) have also devel-oped peripheral neuritis, which appears to be due to a pyridoxine deficiency.

In infants pyridoxine deficiency has been found to produce convulsions possibly due to an inadequate level of γ-aminobutyric acid in the brain.

Nicotinic acid
Nicotinic acid deficiency produces a progressive dementia, with apprehen-sion and confusion in the early stages progressing to severe derangement with maniacal outbursts. In acute nicotinic acid deficiency an encephalo-pathy is found which closely resembles Wernicke's syndrome. This may be accompanied by peripheral neuritis.

Vitamin B_{12}
The characteristic central nervous system lesion of vitamin B_{12} deficiency is subacute combined degeneration of the cord due to demyelination of the dorsal and lateral columns.

Psychosis with mental deterioration has also been reported.

Folic acid
Deficiency of folic acid although producing a megaloblastic bone marrow and macrocytic anaemia, closely resembling, if not identical to, that found in vitamin B_{12} deficiency, is not associated with central nervous system le-sions. However, administration of folic acid to a patient who is deficient in vitamin B_{12} can precipitate a very severe subacute combined degeneration of the cord. Thus, it is important to distinguish between these two causes of a macrocytic anaemia so that the appropriate treatment may be given.

A folic acid deficiency like a deficiency of vitamin B_{12} can produce a psy-chosis.

Vitamin K

In haemorrhagic disease of the new-born associated with vitamin K deficiency a common site for the haemorrhages is into the brain substance or within the cranium so that pressure on the brain results. The exact symptomatology depends upon which part of the brain is damaged.

The blood

Pyridoxine

Pyridoxine deficiency has in certain cases been associated with hypochromic anaemia. In such cases lymphopenia may also be present.

Riboflavine

Rarely riboflavine deficiency produces a microcytic hypochromic anaemia with a hypoplastic marrow.

Biotin

An anaemia may occur in infants with pantothenic acid deficiency but is rare.

Vitamin B_{12}

A deficiency of vitamin B_{12} results in a megaloblastic bone marrow (Plate 11) with a macrocytic anaemia (Plate 10). The polymorphonuclear leucocytes show hypersegmented nuclei.

Folic acid

A macrocytic anaemia with megaloblastic bone marrow is also found with folic acid deficiency.

Ascorbic acid

A moderately severe anaemia is characteristic of scurvy. There has been considerable argument about the cause of this anaemia and in particular whether this is an effect of ascorbic acid on iron transport and haemoglobin production or whether the loss of blood from the haemorrhagic state is the primary cause. Recent evidence suggests that ascorbic acid affects the iron transport mechanism.

Vitamin E

One of the biochemical signs of a vitamin E deficiency is the presence of red cells which are fragile in hydrogen peroxide or dialuric acid. The significance of this finding in relation to the blood within the body is not clear. Tocopherol deficiency leads to a haemolytic anaemia in premature infants.

The heart and the blood vessels

Thiamine

The terminal stage of many patients with thiamine deficiency consists of a circulatory failure due to severely deranged heart muscle. The heart in these patients is grossly enlarged.

The bones

Vitamin A

Although vitamin A deficiency in the majority of experimental and farm animals can produce severe bone changes, none have been reported so far in human vitamin A deficiency.

Vitamin B complex

In animals bone changes can be found with deficiency of pyridoxine, riboflavine and pantothenic acid but no effects on the bones have so far been reported in human deprivation of any member of the B group.

Vitamin D

The characteristic lesions of a vitamin D deficiency are rickets in the young infant and child (Figures 14 to 16) and osteomalacia in the adult. The lesion consists of a failure of the matrix to calcify. Thus the long bones of children show both failure of provisional calcification and of ossification. The cartilage and matrix continue to grow to produce the typical swollen ends of the bones.

Ascorbic acid

The bone lesion of scurvy appears to be due to a failure of development of normal matrix, which does not become ossified in a normal fashion. Irregular masses of calcified cartilage in fibrous tissue occur, marrow spaces become filled with a loose connective tissue and bone shafts are found to be rarefied.

Hypervitaminosis A

Hypervitaminosis A produces bone lesions in both animals and humans. The characteristic picture is found in infants who exhibit painful periosteal thickening over the long bones.

Hypervitaminosis D

Hypervitaminosis D can also produce bony changes. In advanced cases in adults diffuse demineralization of bones is seen, but in infants suffering from the same disease rarefaction of the bones has not so far been described.

The reproductive system

Vitamin deficiencies in most animal species produce extensive changes in both the male and female reproductive organs. Vitamin imbalance during pregnancy in most animal species produces foetal abnormalities.

It is therefore surprising that in the human no clear evidence exists to connect deficiency of any one or more of the vitamins with either reproductive abnormalities or foetal deformities.

Laboratory Tests
for Deficiency

VITAMIN A

Estimation of the degree of vitamin A deficiency can be undertaken by the determination of blood levels for both the vitamin and carotene.

Considerable storage of vitamin A occurs in the body and therefore little correlation exists between the blood level and the true vitamin status in the human. Normal vitamin A levels are usually between 100 and 300 i.u./100 ml and 300 mg/100 ml for carotenoids.

VITAMIN D

Radiology is of great value in the diagnosis of rickets, X-ray examination of the ends of long bones giving the most satisfactory evidence. Measurement of the concentration of the blood alkaline phosphatase level, which rises in rickets, may provide evidence of the disease before X-ray changes can be detected and thus is helpful in the diagnosis of early rickets. It is a non-specific test however. More recently it has been shown that the best diagnostic procedure is the estimation of 25-hydroxycholecalciferol by competitive protein binding.

VITAMIN E

Three tests can be used to determine a tocopherol deficiency state. Serum tocopherol estimation is a reliable index of circulating vitamin. The normal serum level is above 1·0 mg/100 ml although occasional values down to 0·8 mg have been recorded.

Under normal circumstances all the creatine derived from creatine phosphate of muscle is excreted as creatinine. In tocopherol deficiency creatine itself is also excreted in the urine.

Normal red cells are resistant to haemolysis by hydrogen peroxide and dialuric acid but cells from tocopherol-deficient patients show greater sensitivity.

VITAMIN K

There is no direct measurement of vitamin K level in the body. Recognition of vitamin K deficiency depends on the estimation of the levels of the appropriate clotting factors in the serum.

Quick's one stage test is a measure of the 'prothrombin' level and gives a reasonable estimation of the vitamin K status. The thrombotest measures factors VII and IX in addition to prothrombin and is a more reliable guide to the vitamin K depletion state.

ASCORBIC ACID

A deficiency state of ascorbic acid can be determined in several different ways. The significance of some of these methods is discussed elsewhere – page 158.

Plasma levels may be determined by the reduction of 2,6-dichlorophenol-indophenol. Estimation of the ascorbic level of the 'buffy coat' seems to give a reasonable indication of the tissue saturation but the buffy coat estimates both leucocyte and platelet levels. It falls to zero about the time that early signs of scurvy appear. Estimation of true leucocyte levels may be more reliable but is time consuming. The 2,4-dinitrophenyl hydrazine estimation is usually used in this case. It is important to realise that 2,4-dinitrophenyl hydrazine measures both ascorbic acid and dehydroascorbic acid but 2,6-dichlorophenylindophenol only measures ascorbic acid itself.

Single determinations of the urinary excretion of vitamin C are of little or no value as an index of vitamin C nutrition. Some authorities, however, consider that the total output over twenty-four hours gives a reliable indication of the vitamin C content of the tissues. The excretion by an adult of less than 13 to 15 mg per day is said to indicate vitamin C deficiency. The rationale of the saturation test is based on the hypothesis that, following the administration of vitamin C, the surplus is excreted in the urine only when the tissues have become saturated. For careful assessment multiple small doses should be given to avoid overspill from blood levels above the renal threshold. As an approximate guide for bedside and consulting room a simplified saturation method, which requires only one urine estimation, may be employed. Urine passed 4–6 hours after a 300 mg dose of ascorbic acid is collected. Reasonable vitamin C levels are indicated by a characteristic colour change with 2,4-dinitrophenyl hydrazine. A dipstick test has recently been introduced for urinary estimation.

Tests involving the measurement of capillary fragility were extensively used for the detection of vitamin C deficiency. The results have proved inconsistent and the test is now considered to be non-specific unless linked with an ascorbic acid measurement. The intradermal dye test depends upon the power of the vitamin C of the skin to decolorize the blue, 2,6-dichlorophenolindophenol. There is a divergence of opinion as to its value since it is not always possible to correlate the results with those obtained using the excretion test. A recent modification of this test involves the estimation of the rate of loss of colour when a drop of the reagent is placed on the tongue.

VITAMIN B$_1$

The thiamine status of the body can be determined either directly or by estimation of thiamine phosphate dependent enzyme activity.

Several methods have been devised for the estimation of thiamine in body fluids. Plasma levels are so low (0·5–1·3 μg/100 ml) that methods of sufficient sensitivity are not readily available.

The twenty-four hour urine output, one hour fasting excretion and random sample determinations have all been used and are fairly reliable. The best is probably the thiamine excretion per gramme of creatinine in single random urine samples.

Several load tests have ben described and give a reasonable indication of a thiamine deficiency state. An elevation of blood pyruvic acid is observed in thiamine deficiency but the test based on this lacks consistency and specificity. More reliable tests have been devised based on the ratio of lactic acid to pyruvic acid after administration of glucose and after exercise.

Pentose levels in erythrocytes rise during thiamine depletion. The most reliable biochemical evidence of thiamine deficiency for routine laboratory use is a determination of red cell transketolase activity with and without added thiamine pyrophosphate – the so called TPP effect.

VITAMIN B₂

A diagnosis of ariboflavinosis is usually made on the patient's history, clinical examination and response to therapy.

Although microfluorimetric blood estimations have been described, such examinations have not proved very valuable for diagnosis. Erythrocyte riboflavine concentration, (normal values 20–28 μg/100 ml) is chemically more reliable but time-consuming. Moreover, no direct relationship can be found between the red blood cell riboflavine level and the dietary intake, and true clinical cases of ariboflavinosis may show normal blood levels. The determination of erythrocyte glutathione reductase is now regarded as an accurate indication of riboflavine status. A competitive binding estimation of riboflavine has also been described recently using egg protein as substrate.

Urine excretion in single non-timed specimens estimated in terms of creatinine excretion (normal 80–270 μg/g creatinine) are commonly used as load tests of which several have been described. Many factors are associated with variations in excretion (negative nitrogen balance, physical activity, variation in excretion rate in the individual, etc.).

VITAMIN B₆

Several tests are available.

The first of these is the estimation of pyridoxal phosphate in the blood before and after a dose of pyridoxine.

A more reliable estimation of the effective pyridoxal phosphate activity can probably be gained from an estimation of the tryptophan metabolism after tryptophan load. In deficiency states increased amounts of xanthurenic acid are excreted and can be measured.

A recent test involves the estimation of erythrocyte aspartate aminotransferase activity with and without the previous addition of pyridoxal phosphate. Erythrocyte glutamate-oxaloacetate transaminase and glutamate-pyruvate transaminase are also now regarded as useful indications of intracellular pyridoxine activity.

NICOTINIC ACID

It has proved difficult to establish a reliable test to indicate deficiency of nicotinic acid. Blood level determinations do not give an adequate indication. Load tests have been extensively used but the excretion pattern depends on the methylating ability of the patient as well as the intake.

For field surveys, estimation of methyl nicotinic derivatives per gramme of creatinine in random urine samples is probably the most reliable simple test.

VITAMIN B_{12}

A vitamin B_{12} deficiency may be suspected from blood and bone marrow examination (note a folic acid deficiency gives a similar picture). There may on occasions be doubts about the existence of a megaloblastic marrow picture and in such patients an abnormal response to the deoxyuridine suppression of tritiated thymidine by the marrow indicates vitamin B_{12} or folate deficiency.

Estimation of plasma levels may give an indication of the vitamin status but the results are sometimes equivocal.

Blood examination showing macrocytic anaemia, decreased white cell count with oversegmented polymorphonuclear cells and a bilirubin level above the normal value indicate a low vitamin B_{12} or folic acid level. Bone marrow examination reveals a typical megaloblastic picture.

Microbiological estimations of plasma B_{12} level are time consuming but reliable. The organisms most commonly used are *Lactobacillus leishmannii* and *Euglena gracilis*. The normal value is 150–300 $\mu g/ml$.

A vitamin B_{12} absorption test using radioactive labelled B_{12} is now often used in preference to a simple plasma estimation. Radioimmunoassay and isotope dilution techniques are available.

It has recently been suggested that the finding of methylmalonic acid in the urine can be used as an indication of vitamin B_{12} deficiency. The specificity and reliability of this test must await further study.

FOLIC ACID

A diagnosis of folic acid deficiency is normally made on the basis of a macrocytic anaemia and leucopenia, a characteristic megaloblastic marrow (but see comment under vitamin B_{12}) and a normal B_{12} absorption test (above), normal gastric hydrochloric acid, or clinical features which preclude Addisonian pernicious anaemia.

Microbiological measurement of serum folic acid may be undertaken but is difficult, time consuming and sometimes gives equivocal results. The normal value is 5–20 $\mu g/ml$.

A relatively easy test for folic acid deficiency has been described recently. A loading dose of histidine is given. In folic acid deficiency the intermediates of histidine metabolism, urocanic acid, imidazoleacrylic acid or formimino-glutamic acid (FIGLU) are excreted in the urine in increased amounts. The test is, however, non-specific.

PANTOTHENIC ACID

A deficiency of pantothenic acid is usually based on an estimation of the blood pantothenic acid level. Pantothenic acid has also been estimated from co-enzymes A measurements of acetylation activity. Several test substances have been proposed as substrates for acetylation but para-amino benzoic acid is most favoured.

Vitamin Losses in Storage and Preparation of Food

The intake of vitamins into the body calculated from standard tables is rarely accurate. The main reasons for a discrepancy are shown in Table 32.

The normal procedure for vitamin surveys has been to use the values for the raw foods and to reduce them by between 10 and 25 per cent for losses. Such calculated figures normally greatly overstate the true intake.

Table 32 Main causes of discrepancy between vitamin intake based on published figures from standard works and the true vitamin absorption.

Fluctuations in the content of the fresh natural raw food
Presence in any form which cannot be absorbed
Losses during storage
   (a) Natural unprocessed stored food
   (b) Foods processed prior to storage
Losses during food preparation before cooking
Losses during cooking

FLUCTUATION IN THE VITAMIN CONTENT OF THE COMPONENTS OF A MEAL

Wide variations occur in the vitamin content of raw foods depending upon the conditions of feeding, growth, etc. This wide fluctuation is often ignored in the standard tables of food composition. Thus for example the vitamin C content of newly harvested potatoes is about 30 mg per 100 g; this figure falls rapidly to about 8 mg in the spring and continues to fall during storage to virtually nil during the early summer. By using a value of 15 mg per 100 g, a figure which is often quoted, the vitamin content of potatoes is therefore in about 50 per cent of the cases over-estimated even for the raw material.

VITAMIN AVAILABILITY

While chemical analyses give an indication of the total content of vitamins, many of these methods do not assess the availability of the vitamins for absorption. Many of the vitamins are present in a form in which they are not readily available and thus the content as expressed by total composition is not a true indication of biological availability.

Thus for example the ascorbic acid in prepared cabbage is present in the bound form, ascorbinogen, a form which is absorbed very poorly by man.

LOSSES IN STORAGE

The last decade has been a time of great change in the eating habits of industrialized countries. Not only has there been an increase in concentration of the population in cities, but in addition more married women are doubly employed, as wage earners and housewives.

As a result of the increased urbanization, fresh food is usually several days in transit to the kitchen. Moreover there is a marked tendency to use

176

ready prepared foods to avoid the time consuming preparation. Each of the stages of the preparation of food results in losses of vitamins. The vitamin content of the food as eaten is thus the vitamin content of fresh food minus the cumulative losses of the various processes.

Storage of untreated foods

Fruits and vegetables which are harvested a long time before use suffer heavy vitamin losses by enzymatic decomposition. Vitamin C is particularly liable to this type of destruction. In apples stored under domestic conditions the vitamin C content may have fallen to about one-third of the original value after only two to three months. Green vegetables have even greater loss.

Table 33 Effect of length of storage on the vitamin C content of potatoes.

	Ascorbic acid mg/100 g
Main crop freshly dug	30
.. .. stored 1–3 months	20
.. .. .. 4–5 months	15
.. .. .. 6–7 months	10
.. .. .. 8–9 months	8

When stored at room temperature they lose practically all the vitamin C after only a few days but these losses are much less when storage is effected at 0° C. The effect of the length of storage on the vitamin content of potatoes is shown in Table 33.

Storage of treated foods

Blanching

Vegetables are blanched before canning or freezing. Blanching consists of brief exposure to boiling water or steam. For canning this removes gases to ensure vacuum conditions after filling and sealing, and shrinks the material. Its main purpose, however, is to inactivate enzymes which have a detrimental effect during storage. Complete inactivation of enzymes, however, is not normally achieved by blanching, but requires heat sterilization temperature conditions. The losses during blanching depend on the exact conditions. Short exposure to high temperature is less harmful than longer heating at lower temperatures. Estimates that have recently been made suggest that losses due to blanching fluctuate between 13 per cent and 60 per cent for vitamin C; 2 per cent and 30 per cent for thiamine; 5 per cent and 40 per cent for riboflavine. The quoted loss of under 1 per cent for carotene is probably an under estimate for it takes no account of the change of the natural all trans β carotenes to isomers which are not usable by the body for vitamin A synthesis. The vitamin C losses during blanching are caused either by oxidation or by leaching. Thus small vegetables, or pieces with relatively large surface areas lose more ascorbic acid than do larger pieces.

There are probably few differences between steam and water scalding in their effect on the vitamin content.

For the readily oxidizable vitamins (e.g. ascorbic acid and carotene) the loss can be reduced if vegetables are cooled rapidly after blanching. Cooling by cold air is preferable since this reduces the extent of further loss which would result by solution of the vitamin in cold water.

Heat sterilization

The vitamin losses during the process of heat sterilization are generally small because oxygen is excluded during this process. Thiamine is the vitamin most likely to suffer due to its labile nature in heat and considerable thiamine losses have been observed from meat. Heating for a short time at a higher temperature is preferable to the same degree of sterilization produced by longer heating at a lower temperature.

The losses suffered by tinned fruit and meat during sterilization are generally less than those suffered by vegetables, for the acid pH seems to have a protective effect. Only minor losses of riboflavine and nicotinic acid are found during heat sterilization of meat. During the pasteurization of milk variable losses of the vitamins occur depending upon the methods that are used. In general, losses of riboflavine, pyridoxine, pantothenic acid and nicotinic acid are small while greater losses occur in thiamine (10–15 per cent) and ascorbic acid.

Irradiation

There are now many reports on the damage to vitamins caused by food preservation with ionizing radiation. The most sensitive vitamins appear to be thiamine, riboflavine, retinol and tocopherols with nicotinic acid relatively stable.

Freeze drying before irradiation appears to reduce the extent of the loss.

Storage in cans

Once the food has been subjected to its initial preparation and is enclosed in the cans, stability of the vitamins appears to be reasonably good. Thus for example losses of ascorbic acid after storage for two years at 10°C only amounted to some 15 per cent of the initial value. Variations, however, are found depending upon the degree of enzymatic destruction that has occurred during the blanching and sterilization phase.

Aseptic canning

The newer technique of aseptic canning appears to offer no advantage over conventional canning for vitamin stability.

Freezing

Freezing is a very effective method of food preservation for vitamin losses due to chemical decomposition are minimal. In frozen meat stored at low temperatures, thiamine, riboflavine, nicotinic acid and pyridoxine are well retained. It must, however, be appreciated in the case of vegetables that while enzyme decomposition is completely inhibited during the freezing process, rapid decomposition may occur during the thawing and in consequence best results are achieved by rapid blanching prior to the freezing process. This particularly applies to ascorbic acid. The figures in the literature for ascorbic acid losses during deep freezing are very variable, probably depending upon the methods used, but it would seem that a reasonable expectation of loss is 25 per cent of the initial value.

Dehydration

Freeze drying is probably one of the best methods of preservation as far as vitamin retention is concerned, but it is of course not widely practised. Hot air drying of vegetables on the other hand results in a variable but rather high loss in the ascorbic acid, the exact percentage depending upon the conditions used. Under the most favourable conditions probably some 10 to 15 per cent of ascorbic acid is lost by hot air drying of vegetables.

The smoking of fish results in hardly any alteration of the content of those vitamins that have been studied.

Losses of vitamins in the drying of milk are about the same as those found during pasteurization and here again thiamine is the vitamin which suffers most.

FLOUR MILLING

Milling to produce a white flour reduces to a minimum the content of bran and germ. These are valuable sources of most of the factors of the B complex and also of vitamin E while the starchy endosperm is practically devoid of these factors.

Figure 45 shows the calculated losses with various degrees of extraction.

Compulsory or voluntary supplementation of white flour is undertaken in several countries. Vitamins used in the individual countries are considered on page 189.

COOKING

Methods of cooking vary widely from one country to another and even from one part of a country to another and it is only possible to give very broad generalizations. It must, however, be appreciated that data from the literature has little relevance unless the methods used for the preparation of the meal are reasonably similar.

Vegetable preparation

Major losses of the water-soluble vitamins occur in the average kitchen during the preparation of vegetables for cooking. These vegetables are usually washed in large quantities of water as a preliminary stage and in many households are left in the water between the time of preparation and cooking.

In the case of potatoes skinning prior to cooking removes a large proportion of the ascorbic acid.

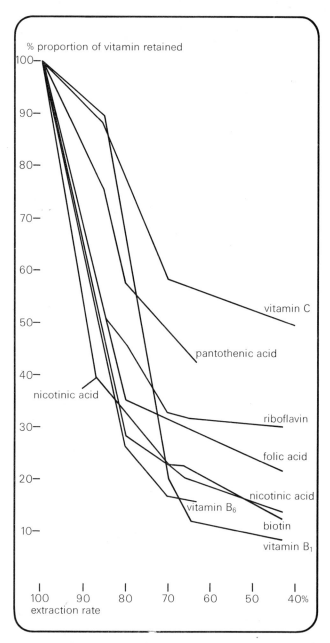

Figure 45 Proportion of vitamins retained compared with the extraction rate of flour. Based on data from T. Moran 'Nutrition Abstracts and Reviews, 29.1.1959'.

180

vitamins	daily requirements	200 g of unenriched white bread (70% extract) percentage of daily requirements supplied	200 g of whole wheat bread (95% extract) percentage of daily requirements supplied
B₁	1·2 mg	10%	50%
B₂	1·8 mg	2%	14%
PP	15·0 mg	8%	40%
Iron	15·0 mg	12%	30%

Figure 46 Bread as a source of vitamins. Vitamins contained in 200 g of bread. From 'Schweiz. Lebensmittelbuch' vol. 1, 5th edition, 1960.

While some of these losses during the course of preparation are largely avoidable, the methods used are so ingrained that re-education would be a major problem.

Baking

Nicotinic acid and riboflavine are almost unaffected in the baking of bread, but losses of thiamine amount to some 25 per cent. The method of baking seems to have very little effect on these losses, but brown bread shows a greater percentage loss than does white (Figure 46).

Cooking

Some of the principles outlined above in relation to methods of industrial preparation of food can also be applied in general terms to cooking within the household. Thus for example slow long cooking and slow cooling, especially with exposure to oxygen brings about more vitamin losses than does rapid heating, cooking and cooling, as for example in a pressure cooker. However, even with the best methods, losses of about 50 per cent can be expected for some of the less stable vitamins and particularly those that are water soluble (e.g. ascorbic acid).

In the case of meat, riboflavine and nicotinic acid are relatively stable and losses average about 10 per cent. The chief losses occur for thiamine, pyridoxine and pantothenic acid where losses of 50 per cent are not uncommon.

Microwave cooking

The vitamin losses from electronic cooking by microwave heating compare closely with those that result from conventional cooking methods.

OVERALL LOSSES

The losses during the processes of food preparation are cumulative and theoretical values can be obtained from a study of the individual processes involved during the preparation. However, the exact conditions vary so much that it is probably important to study the final food product rather than calculate the value from anticipated losses from the various procedures.

The variability of the individual losses depending upon the method of processing is shown in Figure 47.

IDEAL COOKING PROCEDURES TO RETAIN THE VITAMIN CONTENT OF NATURAL FOODS

From what has been said in the preceding paragraphs it may be concluded that ideal food preparation and cooking methods for the preservation of vitamin content are as follows:

Use fresh food as opposed to stored food.

Minimum amount of water used in their preparation.

Minimum cooking, and where cooking is essential a high temperature for a short time is probably preferable.

No storage of cooked foods prior to eating.

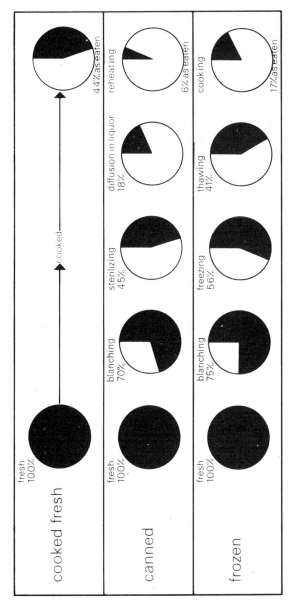

Percentage retention of vitamin C during the processing and cooking of peas treated in different ways.

While these are the ideals, modern urban life makes them difficult to achieve. In addition palatability is an important consideration for food preparation. Preparation of dishes which are the delight of the gourmet are rarely compatible with these principles of maintenance of vitamin content.

STABILITY TO PROCESSING IN THE INDIVIDUAL VITAMINS

Vitamin A

The sensitivity of vitamin A to oxygen and light suggests that much of the activity contained in foods would be lost during storage and preparation. Experiments indicate that there is indeed loss at high temperatures in the presence of oxygen but generally both vitamin A and provitamin A carotenoids demonstrate good stability in food processing.

Vitamin D

Vitamin D is resistant to oxidation in the air, even up to 100°C. No changes occur with alkalis.

In the normal household and factory preparation and preservation of food, no loss of activity is likely to occur.

Vitamin E

Accurate quantitative determinations of tocopherol in foods has only recently been possible and data in the literature is often misleading. Tocopherols are sensitive to oxidation, particularly in the presence of heat and alkalis. Recent studies have shown a fairly serious degradation of alpha-tocopherol in frozen foods. Cooking food in large amounts of fat may destroy 70-90 per cent of the tocopherol. The greatest losses occur when rancid fats and oils are used for cooking; even a degree of rancidity which cannot be tasted suffices for quantitative destruction of vitamin E. Bleaching of flour completely destroys vitamin E. Baking itself incurs losses which are not very great and other losses in preparation keep within tolerable limits.

Vitamin K

The vitamin is sensitive to acids, alkalis, oxidizing agents, light and ultraviolet radiation. In particular, it is thought that this vitamin can easily be destroyed by ionizing rays.

Vitamin C

Even immediately after being harvested, the crops can lose a considerable amount of their vitamin C as a result of processing and cooking (Table 34).

The primary reason for ascorbic acid loss is that it can be readily oxidized particularly in the presence of traces of heavy metal.

Milk suffers losses of ascorbic acid which amounts generally to a third and often a half or two-thirds as a result of pasteurizing, sterilizing, condensing and drying. A similar situation exists for the drying and sterilizing

Table 34 Losses of ascorbic acid during various food preparation methods (expressed in terms of percentage remaining).

	Ascorbic acid
Potatoes	
fresh dug main crop	30 mg/100 g
boiled, peeled	50–70% raw value
in jacket, baked	80% raw value
Milk	
whole raw	2·0 mg/100 g
pasteurized	75% raw value
Cabbage	
raw	60 mg/100 g
cooked	33% raw value
Frozen vegetables	75% raw value
Canned vegetables	85–40% raw value

of fruit and vegetables. The secondary reason for losses of vitamin C is its ready solubility in water.

Heat is the primary cause of diminished amounts of ascorbic acid because it accelerates the course of the oxidation and extraction processes. To protect the vitamin C, therefore, warm storage and re-heating should be avoided. It can be said in general that the extent of the losses depends very largely upon the details of the preparation so that the losses vary very much from one household to another.

Vitamin B_1

Thiamine can easily be removed during the preparation of foods, both by leaching and by removal of those parts of the raw foodstuff where the vitamin B_1 is concentrated. Polished rice and white flour form poor sources unless the vitamin content has been artificially restored.

Apart from the two causes of vitamin B_1 impoverishment mentioned above, this vitamin can also be destroyed by heat; in the baking of bread, 15–25 per cent may be lost compared with the dough; according to one examination the loss in the crust was 30 per cent and that in the rest 7 per cent; rusks, baked twice, lost 40–50 per cent.

According to the method of cooking, lamb loses 30–50 per cent of its vitamin B_1 content and veal and beef 25–75 per cent. Milk loses up to a third of its content in the sterilizing process. Since vitamin B_1 is sensitive to alkalis, the addition of baking soda when cooking vegetables has a particularly bad effect.

Vitamin B_2

As might be expected from the marked fluorescence, riboflavine is sensitive to light. Milk which is exposed to light in summer, loses 90 per cent of its content of B_2 in full sunshine within two hours, 45 per cent in cloudy weather and 30 per cent when the sky is completely clouded over. Under mild conditions – say, the light intensity in a room – one must still reckon on a 30 per cent loss within 24 hours.

Hardly any losses occur, on the other hand, if the food is stored in the dark, especially if it has an acid reaction; after 48 days in cold storage, beef showed the same content of riboflavine as immediately after slaughter.

Heating produces small losses. The loss is estimated at 12–25 per cent in the case of boiled milk and about 14 per cent on pasteurization. The losses in the preparation of meat are of much the same order. The simultaneous influence of light will increase these losses during cooking.

Losses of vitamin B_2 during preparation depend on the quantity of water used and the length of soaking.

Vitamin B_6

The greatest loss of vitamin B_6 probably results from its being washed out during food preparation. It is considered stable to heat, oxygen and acids; yet losses were found when meat was roasted, amounting to, on average, half the original content. Milk loses one to two-thirds of its vitamin B_6 during sterilization. Vegetables preserved in tins can also lose up to 80 per cent of their content of vitamin B_6, the part which passes into the liquid not being counted as a loss.

Nicotinic acid (Niacin)

Nicotinic acid is stable in the presence of atmospheric oxygen, acids, light and heat and also has a marked resistance to ionizing radiation. In normal food preparation, nicotinic acid is hardly destroyed at all although it can be washed out by water, e.g. during blanching when up to 40 per cent of the nicotinic acid content is lost. None is lost in the pasteurization and sterilization of milk or in the production of dried milk or dried egg.

Vitamin B_{12}

Light and ultraviolet rays rapidly destroy vitamin B_{12} in pure solution, although losses are small in milk.

As in the case of all water soluble vitamins significant losses can occur by leaching during food preparation.

Pantothenic acid

Wheat suffers a loss of approximately 60 per cent during manufacturing processes, meat 30 per cent loss during cooking. There is a small loss with vegetable preparation. Apart from this, food preparation and cooking does not seem to cause much loss of pantothenic acid.

Addition of Vitamins to Food

Attention has already been drawn to the changing pattern of our dietary habits over the past ten to twenty-five years, resulting from the increase in urban life and the habit of married women undertaking other jobs in addition to their housework. In consequence of these changed dietary habits the vitamin content of food as actually consumed has fallen markedly from the days when fresh food was taken and prepared straight from the garden. Details of the causes and extent of these losses are given on pages 176 to 186.

It is now appreciated that the losses of vitamins during the processing of foods reduce the intake so much that some people are in danger of receiving inadequate amounts of vitamins to maintain normal health.

In consequence in nearly all countries it is now the established practice to add vitamins to appropriate items of the diet with the intention of ensuring that the minimal requirements for normal health are achieved by the majority of the population. In most countries this addition of vitamins to the food is carefully controlled by the appropriate governmental authority and maximum levels are defined.

In some countries the addition of vitamins to certain items of food is compulsory, but in the majority the addition of vitamins is still on a voluntary basis. It is important to appreciate that this addition of vitamins can be undertaken in different ways and different terminology is employed for the various procedures:

Re-vitaminization — restoring the vitamin content to that originally present before processing occurred.

Standardization — compensating for natural variation in the vitamin content.

Enrichment — adding more than the amount of the vitamin already present.

Vitaminization — food as carriers of vitamins which are not normally present.

VITAMIN RESTORATION

The best example of vitamin restoration is that of white flour. Wheat represents a valuable source of vitamins (Figure 46). However, as has been demonstrated, the extraction of the darker outer layers by milling to produce a white flour removes a large proportion of these vitamins and the extent depends upon the degree of extraction (Figure 45). Attempts to repopularize wholemeal products seemed doomed to failure and in consequence a process of vitamin restoration is now undertaken in many countries. It has been estimated that some 250 million people in the Western World eat bread which has had vitamins added and these vitamins undoubtedly play an important part in the maintenance of an adequate daily intake.

While it would probably be desirable to restore the wheat entirely to its whole state this is not normally undertaken and only the more important components are added. The extent of this restoration process varies from one country to another and in some an attempt is made at supplementation.

The figures for the quantities of the vitamins and minerals added to white flour in various countries is shown in Table 35.

Similar conditions apply in those countries where rice forms the staple item of diet. Milling of the rice also removes most of the vitamin content. In certain areas vitamin restoration of rice is already being undertaken.

Table 35 Recommended additions for wheat flour of low extraction rate in mg/kg of flour.

Country	Thiamine	Riboflavine	Niacin	Calcium	Iron
Brazil	4·50	2·50	—	970	30·0
Canada	4·18	2·42	30·5	500	26·0—37·0
Denmark	5·00	5·00	—	800	30·0
Germany	3·00—4·00	1·50—5·00	20·0	—	—
Great Britain	2·40	—	16·0	480	16·5
Sweden	2·60—4·00	1·20	23·0—40·0	—	11·0
Switzerland	4·18	2·53	50·0	—	26·4
USA	4·18	2·42—2·53	30·5	290	10·0—13·0
USSR	4·00	4·00	20·0	—	—

More recently, the production of dehydrated potato for 'instant mash' which may result in the total destruction of vitamin C in the finished material, has called for the addition of ascorbic acid to restore the product to its original full content.

STANDARDIZATION AND ENRICHMENT
While the process of restoration is now fairly widely accepted, that of standardization of preparations or enrichment above the natural level is not so widely practised. Indeed in some countries it is not permitted by law. Examples of standardization and enrichment can be found in the case of vitamin C in fruit juices and vitamin A in milk.

VITAMINIZATION
The main object of vitaminization is to take a widely used and relatively inexpensive commodity and to incorporate in this sufficient vitamins to cover the needs of the majority of the population. Margarine is a typical example. This product, produced predominantly from vegetable oils, contains practically no vitamins A or D and has been used as a carrier for both these vitamins in many countries. The amount of these vitamins added varies from one country to another. In some cases this is controlled by law, in others it is a voluntary arrangement. In addition to vitamin additions, some margarines are now being produced which contain added quantities of essential fatty acids. As shown previously (page 62) essential fatty acids in large amounts increase the vitamin E requirements and there is a case for adding α-tocopherol to such margarines.

A recent development is the production of new foods from cheap local raw materials having an adequate content of high grade protein. Since these are primarily intended for use in areas where malnutrition is rife, extensive vitamin enrichment of these products is obviously desirable.

Vitamins in Animal Feeds

The change in the practice of animal husbandry over the last few years has been no less dramatic than alterations in the pattern of human eating habits. Intensive breeding for rapid growth and maximum feed conversion is now the rule rather than the exception. The animals are now often confined rather than being allowed to gather most of their own food. The quantity and quality of feed is continually being improved. Housing and modern hygiene are now of a high standard. As a consequence of these new methods considerable improvements in yields have been achieved. (Figure 48).

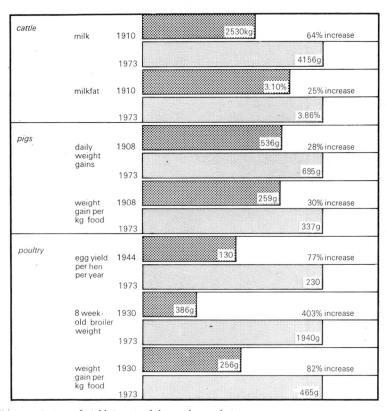

Figure 48 Improved yields in animals by modern techniques.

Among the factors which have made these changes possible has been the greater use of supplementary vitamins in the diet, for stored feed, like stored human food, is grossly vitamin deficient (Figure 49). During recent years the vitamin requirements of the various species of animals have been studied very extensively. Table 36 summarizes the present estimated requirements based on the findings. These figures represent the average vitamin requirement for optimum growth, yield and fertility under normal conditions. If the conditions are not normal (adverse surroundings, dis-

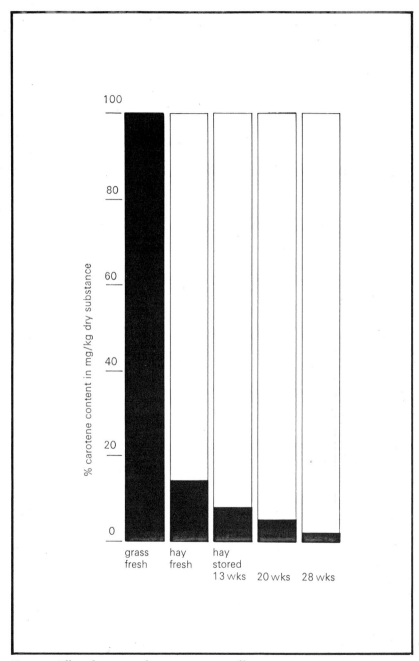

Figure 49 Effect of storage on the carotene content of hay.

Table 36 Vitamin requirements of various animal species. Expressed as quantities per kg of ration unless otherwise stated.

Vitamin / Quantities per kg of ration (about 90% dry matter)	A	D_3	E	K	B_1	B_2	Nicotinic acid	Pantothenic acid	B_6	B_{12}	Folic acid	Biotin	Choline	C
	I.U.	I.U.	I.U.	mg	mg	mg	mg	mg	mg	mg	mg	mg	mg	mg
POULTRY														
Chicks and broilers (starting)	15,000	1,500	30	3	3	8	50	20	7	0·030	1·5	0·15	1,500	60
Chicks and broilers (growing)	10,000	1,000	25	2	3	6	40	12	5	0·020	0·7	0·10	1,300	60
Hens, Ducks (laying and breeding)	12,000	1,200	30	2	3	6	40	15	5	0·010	1·5	0·20	1,100	50
Turkey (starting)	15,000	1,500	35	3	3	8	80	20	7	0·020	1·5	0·35	2,000	60
Turkey (growing and fattening)	10,000	1,100	30	2	3	6	70	15	5	0·015	1·5	0·20	1,700	60
Turkey (breeding)	12,000	1,200	40	2	3	8	70	25	6	0·015	1·5	0·30	1,700	50
PIGS														
Piglets (starting)	15,000	1,500	30	3	3	6	25	20	6	0·04		0·20	1,200	300
Pigs (growing)	10,000	1,000	25	1	2·5	5	20	15	5	0·03		0·15	1,000	
Pigs (fattening)	5,000	500	20	0·5	2	4	15	13	4	0·02		0·10	900	150
Sows (breeding)	12,000	1,200	25	1	2·5	6	15	12	5	0·02		0·22	900	

Table 36 (continued)

Vitamin Quantities per kg of ration (about 90% dry matter)	A	D₃	E	K	B₁	B₂	Nicotinic acid	Pantothenic acid	B₆	B₁₂	Folic acid	Biotin	Choline	C
	I.U.	I.U.	I.U.	mg	mg	mg	mg	mg	mg	mg	mg	mg	mg	mg
RUMINANTS														
Calves (0–3 months)*	20,000	2,000	40		4	7	25	12	5	0·02		0·10	400	500†
Cattle (rearing)**	25,000	3,000	150											
Cattle (fattening)**	40,000	5,000	250											
Dairy cows**	50,000	8,000	350											
Sheep and goats**	4,000	250	25											
HORSES														
Foals	10,000	1,500	50		6	10	30	12	3	0·03	3		150	
Yearlings	20,000	3,000	100		12	20	60	25	6	0·06	6		300	
Working and saddle horses	40,000	6,000	300		20	40	100	40	10	0·10	10		450	
Race horses and breeding horses	40,000	6,000	1,000		30	50	120	50	15	0·15	15		600	
OTHERS														
Dogs	10,000	1,000	40		3	5	25	10	3	0·03	0·3	0·25	1,000	
Cats	18,000	1,800	50		8	8	60	12	6	0·02	0·4	0·25	1,500	
Rabbits	9,000	900	40		2	6	50	20	2	0·01			1,300	
Mink and foxes	10,000	1,000	80		4	6	30	15	2	0·03	0·6	0·25	1,000	
Fish (trout)	8,000	1,000	125	15	10	25	200	50	15	0·02	4·0	1·00	1,500	450

* per day per 100 kg live weight.   ** per day per animal.   † 500 daily for the first two weeks.

ease and other forms of stress) the daily doses must be increased accordingly. Under certain conditions the vitamin requirements can indeed be several times greater than these specified values. Since the majority of animal feeding practices are based on manufactured compound feeds, vitamin enrichment is easily and inexpensively achieved by adding the appropriate quantity of synthetic vitamins shown in Table 36 (page 194).

Index

Printed in Great Britain by R. & R. Clark Ltd, Edinburgh